FOREWORD

WILLIAM OSLER brought to modern medicine an insistence on accuracy, completeness and deference that are the qualities around which a successful clinical encounter is achieved. No doctor ever ceases to learn and become more competent in the processes of history taking and the skills of physical examination. Summarising a problem for the patient and relatives, communicating with colleagues and ensuring the best possible outcome as the advocate of the patient are the essence of clinical practice.

In taking the first steps along this challenging path the new student of medicine is confronted by a daunting series of unknowns and must enter a learning process as quickly as possible. Each new skill acquired helps in the acquisition of others and adds to confidence and satisfaction.

A medical life is built around personal encounters, and communication skills must be constantly refined. As the student progresses through the process of clinical history taking, physical examination and reporting and recording, this book will provide a solid foundation. It will be used frequently at first and later become a valued support as the steps become second nature and diagnosis and treatment come to be dominant issues. Carry this book in your pocket to wards and clinics, observe the techniques of experienced clinicians and evolve for yourself the confidence in your clinical skills that is one of the great rewards of a practising life.

Peter Castaldi

Professor of Medicine
The University of Sydney

PREFACE

Physical Examination is ordinarily taken to mean
examination of the patient using the examiner's
five senses aided only by the portable tools of his
trade such as stethoscope, tendon hammer,
ophthalmoscope etc . . .

THE OXFORD MEDICAL COMPANION 1994

*The distance doesn't matter; it is only the first step
that is difficult.*

MARQUISE DE DEFFOND (1697–1780)

When junior medical students first enter the wards, they are expected to start mastering history taking and physical examination immediately. They may be faced with patients who have problems in all areas of medicine. Moreover, those undertaking the new 4-year graduate medical program will be expected to examine patients when they have at first only minimal background knowledge. It is difficult for the student beginning work in the wards to remember all of the relevant details when performing history taking and physical examination.

With experience and practice, students will develop their own systematic approaches to examination but at the start specific guidance is essential. This book provides an introduction to history taking and the examination of patients for first-time students, giving step by step instructions. We were encouraged to write it, in part because our students have complained that our larger book, *Clinical Examination: A Guide to Physical Diagnosis*, would not fit comfortably into their coat pockets. This book should fit into almost anyone's white coat pocket. It has been written to complement *Clinical Examination* directly.

We have designed this pocket book to fulfill students' needs. It is meant to be carried around in the wards and referred to constantly. The book deals first with history taking and with physical examination of the regions of the body: examination of the major systems is then summarised. Details of the mechanisms of symptoms and signs, and comprehensive lists of differential diagnosis are not included here but are available in *Clinical Examination*.

We hope that this *Pocket Edition of Clinical Examination* will assist medical students to learn and remember the key aspects of history taking and physical examination that they will then need to apply for the rest of their medical careers.

Nicholas J Talley
Simon O'Connor

Sydney and Canberra
January, 1998

ACKNOWLEDGMENTS

'Specialist — A man who knows more and more about less and less.'

WILLIAM JAMES MAYO (1861–1934)

We are grateful to the following specialists who have reviewed sections of this book. We take responsibility for any errors or omissions.

Dr M Dally FRACP, Consultant Respiratory Physician, Nepean Hospital, Sydney.

Dr A Fitzpatrick MD, FRACP, Clinical Senior Lecturer in Medicine, University of Sydney, Director of Cardiology, Nepean Hospital, Sydney.

Dr B Frankum FRACP, Lecturer in Medical Education, University of Sydney and Staff Specialist in Immunology Nepean Hospital, Sydney.

Dr P McManis MD, FRACP, Senior Lecturer in Medicine, University of Sydney and Staff Specialist in Neurology, Nepean Hospital, Sydney.

Dr T Shakeshaft FRACS, Lecturer in Surgery, University of Sydney, Nepean Hospital, Sydney.

Professor J Wiley MD, FRACP, Professor of Haematology. University of Sydney, Nepean Hospital, Sydney.

CONTENTS

CHAPTER 1

Taking the history and beginning the examination

When you hear hoofbeats,
think of horses not zebras.

THE ZEBRA RULE

THE HISTORY

Unlike veterinary surgeons and to some extent paediatricians, adult doctors can usually deduce a reasonable differential diagnosis (a list of the possible diagnoses, suggested by a set of symptoms or signs) simply by talking to the patient. Remember that symptoms are subjective feelings perceptible to the patient while signs are changes that can be demonstrated objectively. Even when the possible diagnoses are not clear after the history has been taken, the likely region or system of the body that is affected will usually be obvious. This enables the clinician to direct the examination appropriately. Except for patients who are extremely ill, the taking of a careful medical history should precede both examination and treatment. Taking the history and examining the patient are also, of course, the least expensive ways of making a diagnosis.

BEDSIDE MANNER

The word 'clinical' is derived from the Greek word meaning *'of or pertaining to a bed'* (*Oxford English Dictionary*, 2nd Edn). The

1

rather old-fashioned term *bedside manner* therefore seems appropriate for describing the clinician's approach to the patient. A professional manner will make history taking and physical examination enjoyable and rewarding for both the student doctor and the patient. This is not an easy skill to describe or teach but should be learnt at the bedside by observing the methods (both successful and unsuccessful) of senior colleagues.

At the end of the interview and examination the clinician must explain as clearly as possible to the patient what the clinical diagnosis is and what this means. The explanation must include discussion of the prognosis (likely outcome of the illness) and the investigations, treatment and the probable length of hospital stay that are to be recommended to the patient. Remember that the clinician's recommendations are just that; it should be clear to patients that they can freely accept or reject them (except in the most unusual circumstances). A clinician whose recommendations are rejected by his or her patient has probably made a poor attempt at explaining them.

Patients should be asked at the end of the assessment if they have any questions and if there are any close relatives or friends who should be involved in the discussion.

For confused or forgetful patients, including some elderly patients, the history may be better obtained partly or completely via a suitable family member or close friend. For patients who speak little English, use of an official medical interpreter or bilingual relative may be appropriate. The interposition of a relative or interpreter between the clinician and the patient always makes the history taking less direct and the patient's symptoms more subject to 'filtering' or interpretation before the information reaches the clinician.

OBTAINING THE HISTORY

The medical interview deals not only with the organic problems of the patient but also with psychosocial aspects of the illness. Good history taking improves the accuracy and completeness of the medical diagnosis and promotes the doctor-patient relationship. In order to develop an effective interviewing technique, the clinician must make a conscious effort to listen to the patient and to establish rapport.

It is useful to make rough notes while questioning the patient. At the end of the history and examination a detailed record is made. This record must be a sequential, accurate account of the development and course of the illness or illnesses of the patient.

A systematic approach to history taking and recording is the most reliable way to avoid missing crucial information (Table 1.1). At the end, the record must make it clear whether the patient's problem is one of diagnosis (i.e., what is wrong) or of management (i.e., what tests and treatment are necessary), or both.

TABLE 1.1   History Taking Sequence

Presenting (Principal) Symptom (PS)

History of Presenting Illness (HPI)
Details of current illnesses and treatments
Details of previous similar episodes
Psychological medical history
Extent of functional disability

Past History (PH)
Past illnesses and surgical operations
Past treatments and drug allergies
Blood transfusions
Menstrual and reproductive history for women

Social History (SH)
Occupation, education
Smoking, alcohol, analgesic abuse
Overseas travel
Marital status
Living conditions

Family History (FH)

Systems Review (SR)

▉ INTRODUCTORY QUESTIONS

Introduce yourself to the patient. It is important here to address the patient respectfully and use his or her name and title. It is usually sufficient to introduce yourself as a student doctor.

In order to obtain a good history the clinician must interview in a **logical manner**, **listen** carefully, **interrupt** appropriately, note **non-verbal clues**, establish a **good relationship** and **correctly interpret** the information obtained.

The clinician should sit down beside the patient so as to be close to eye level and give the impression that the interview will be an unhurried one. The next step should be to **find out the patient's major complaint or complaints**. It is best to attempt a conversational approach and ask 'What has been the trouble or problem recently?' or 'When did these problems begin?' If the patient has already been interviewed by the resident, the registrar, the consultant and three medical students it may be necessary to apologise and explain the importance of hearing about the problem again in the patient's own words. **Allow the patient to tell the whole story, then ask questions to fill in the gaps.**

To ensure the best possible communication between the patient and doctor it is important to try to make the patient feel comfortable. You should try to appear (and to feel) relaxed and not in a hurry, even if it is lunch time. Appropriate (but not exaggerated) reassuring gestures may be useful. If the patient stops giving the story spontaneously, it can be useful to provide a short summary of what has already been said and encourage the patient to continue.

The clinician must learn to listen with an open mind. The temptation to leap to specific questions before the patient has had the chance to describe all the symptoms in his or her own words should be resisted. However, some direction may be necessary to keep a talkative patient on track later during the interview. Avoid using pseudo-medical terms and if the patient uses these, find out exactly what is meant by them as misinterpretation of medical terms is common.

'Sympathetic confrontation' can be helpful in some situations. For example, if the patient appears sad, angry or frightened, referring to this in a tactful way may lead to the volunteering of appropriate information.

Some patients may have medical problems that make the interview difficult for them; these include deafness and problems with speech and memory. These must be recognised by the clinician if the interview is to be successful.

 # THE PRESENTING (PRINCIPAL) SYMPTOM

An attempt must be made to decide which of the patient's symptoms (there may be more than one) led the patient to present. It must be remembered that the patient's and the doctor's idea of what constitutes a serious problem may differ. Record each presenting symptom in the patient's own words, avoiding technical terms. Later on the symptoms should be recorded in a more formal medical format.

It is suggested that the history be taken in the following order but using open-ended questions where possible.

CURRENT SYMPTOMS AND HISTORY OF THE PRESENTING ILLNESS

Let the patient describe the symptoms that have caused him or her to seek medical help. Quite a lot of detail about the course and nature of all the symptoms is required. When the history of the presenting illness is written down, the events should be placed in chronological order or, if numerous systems are affected, in chronological order for each system. As set out below, certain information should routinely be sought for each of the symptoms, if this hasn't been volunteered by the patient.

Time Course

Find out when the symptom first began and try to date this as accurately as possible. A patient asked 'How long has this pain been present?' will not uncommonly say, 'for a long time, doctor'. It is necessary then, if the interview is not to be rather tedious, to ask 'Do you mean a few hours or many weeks?' Although one should not suggest answers to the patient, giving a few possible alternatives may speed things up.

Mode of Onset and Pattern

Find out whether the symptom came on rapidly, gradually or instantaneously at the date of onset. Certain symptoms are typically of very sudden onset (like turning on a light), for example, the onset of a fast heartbeat in supraventricular tachycardia. Ask whether the symptom has been present continuously or intermittently. Determine if the symptom is getting worse or better, and if so, when the change occurred. Some symptoms are at their very worst at the moment of onset (e.g., the pain of aortic dissection). Find out what the patient was doing at the time the symptom began.

Site and Radiation

Ask where the symptom is exactly and whether it is localised or diffuse. Ask the patient to point to the actual site on the body. Also determine if the symptom, if localised, radiates (travels elsewhere). The pattern of radiation is very suggestive of certain abnormalities, for example, the distribution of pain and paraesthesiae (pins and needles) in the territory of the median nerve of the hand in carpal tunnel syndrome. Other symptoms such as cough, dyspnoea (shortness of breath), change in weight or dizziness are not localised.

Character

Here it is necessary to ask the patient what is meant by the symptom. If the patient complains of dizziness, does this mean the room spins around (vertigo) or is it more a feeling of lightheadedness? It may be necessary to suggest some alternative descriptions; for example, a patient may find chest discomfort difficult to describe. It is reasonable then to ask if the feeling is tight, heavy, sharp or stabbing. It is interesting to note that patients who have been stabbed do not usually describe the pain as stabbing.

Severity

This is subjective. The best way to assess severity is to ask the patient if the symptom interferes with normal activities or sleep. It is often suggested that patients be asked to give the symptom (usually in this case pain) a number between 0 and 10, where 10 represents the most severe pain the patient has ever experienced and 0 represents no pain. It is simpler to ask if the symptom is very mild, moderate, severe or very severe.

Aggravating or Relieving Factors

Ask if anything makes the symptom worse or better. For example, lying flat may make the dyspnoea of heart failure worse but not that of chronic airflow limitation (chronic bronchitis or emphysema).

Associated Symptoms and Factors

Here an attempt is made to uncover in a systematic way symptoms which might be expected to be associated with a particular disease or risk factors that make the disease more likely. For example a strong family history of carcinoma of the colon makes rectal bleeding a more sinister symptom. A patient who presents with cardiac symptoms must have the major risk factors for coronary artery disease (e.g., smoking and family history) assessed in detail.

CURRENT TREATMENT

Ask the patient if he or she is currently taking any tablets or medicines. Attempt to find out the names and doses of each. Remember that non-prescription drugs may not be thought relevant and may have to be asked about specifically. Always ask if a woman is taking a contraceptive pill, because it is not considered a medicine or tablet by many who take it.

MENSTRUAL HISTORY

A menstrual history should always be obtained for women; it is particularly relevant for a patient with abdominal pain, a suspected endocrine disease or genitourinary symptoms. Write down the date of the last menstrual period. Ask about the age at which menstruation began, if the periods are regular, or whether menopause has occurred. Do not forget to ask a woman in the childbearing years if there is a possibility of pregnancy; this, for example, may preclude the use of certain investigations (e.g., involving X-rays) or drugs.

PSYCHOLOGICAL MEDICINE HISTORY

Any medical illness may affect the psychological status of a patient. Moreover, pre-existing psychological factors may influence the way a medical problem presents. Psychiatric disease can also present with medical symptoms. Therefore, an essential part of the history taking process is to obtain information about psychological distress and the mental state. A sympathetic unhurried approach using open-ended questions will provide much information that can then be systematically recorded after the interview. It is important for the history taker to maintain an objective demeanour, particularly when asking about delicate subjects such as sexual problems, grief reactions or abuse.

The formal psychological or psychiatric interview differs from general medical history taking. It takes considerable time for patients to develop rapport with, and confidence in, the interviewer. There are certain standard questions that may give valuable insights into the patient's state of mind (Tables 1.2, 1.3 and 1.4). It may be important to obtain much more detailed information about each of these issues, depending on the clinical circumstances. Discussion of sensitive issues may actually be therapeutic in some cases.

TABLE 1.2 Personal History

USEFUL QUESTIONS TO ASK:

Where do you live (e.g., a house, flat, or hostel?).

Tell me about your current work and where you have worked in the past.

TABLE 1.2   Continued

USEFUL QUESTIONS TO ASK:

Do you get on well with people at home?

Do you get on well with people at work?

Do you have any financial problems?

Are you married or have you been married?

Could you tell me about your close relationships?

Would you describe your marriage (or living arrangements) as happy?

Would you say you have a large number of friends?

Are you religious?

Do you feel you are too fat or too thin?

Has anyone in the family had problems with psychiatric illness?

Have you ever had a nervous breakdown?

Have you ever had any psychiatric problem?

TABLE 1.3   Symptoms of Depression

USEFUL QUESTIONS TO ASK:

Have you been feeling sad, down or blue?

Have you felt depressed or lost interest in things daily for 2 or more weeks in the past?

Have you ever felt like taking your own life?

Have you had early morning wakening?

Has your appetite been poor recently?

Have you lost weight recently?

How do you feel about the future?

Have you had trouble concentrating on things?

Have you had guilty thoughts?

Have you lost interest in things you usually enjoy?

TABLE 1.4   Symptoms of Anxiety

USEFUL QUESTIONS TO ASK:

Do you worry excessively about things?

Do you have trouble relaxing?

Do you have problems getting to sleep at night?

Do you feel uncomfortable in crowded places?

Do you worry excessively about minor things?

Do you feel suddenly frightened or anxious or panicky for no reason is situations in which most people would not be afraid?

Do you find you have to do things repetitively such as washing your hands multiple times?

Do you have any rituals (such as checking things) that you feel you have to do, even though you know it may be silly?

Do you have recurrent thoughts that you have trouble controlling?

While the patient is describing the symptoms, make observations to help you draw inferences about his or her personality. For example, dress, facial expressions, (e.g., the amount of distress while describing personal issues), signs of anxiety or restlessness, and mannerisms should be noted as you discuss issues with the patient.

THE EFFECT OF THE ILLNESS

Any serious or chronic illness may cause severe financial or social problems that should be explored and documented. These need to be taken into account when planning the best treatment.

THE PAST HISTORY

Next, aspects of the patient's past history that have not yet emerged must be sought systematically.

PAST ILLNESSES

Ask the patient if there have been any serious illnesses or operations or admissions to hospital in the past and at what age these occurred. Find out about serious illnesses in childhood that interfered with school. It is often necessary to ask how a particular diagnosis was made in the past, as the patient's impression of what was wrong may not be correct.

A history of multiple accidents or serious illnesses may suggest another underlying problem. For example, alcohol or drug abuse may be the cause of repeated motor accidents or head injuries. Elderly patients may have multiple falls because of neurological or bone disease.

PAST TREATMENT AND ALLERGIC HISTORY

There are some medications or treatments the patient may have had in the past which remain relevant; these include corticosteroids, oral contraceptives, antihypertensive agents, blood transfusions and chemotherapy or radiotherapy for malignancy.

Note any adverse reactions which have occurred in the past. One should also ask about any allergy to drugs, and what the allergic reaction actually involved. Often the patient confuses an allergy with the side effect of a drug.

Determine the immunisation status (DPT, rubella, polio, mumps, measles, influenza, *Haemophilus influenzae* and hepatitis B). Ask about past screening tests such as Papanicolaou's smear, mammography, chest X-rays, stool occult blood testing or sigmoidoscopy.

THE SOCIAL AND PERSONAL HISTORY

This history includes the whole economic, social, domestic and industrial situation of the patient. Ask first about the place of birth and residence. Ask patients to list who is at home with them in order to ascertain marital status or other living arrangements, and the home environment. Determine the level of education obtained. Race is important in some diseases, such as thalassaemia and sickle cell anaemia.

OCCUPATION

Ask the patient about his or her present occupation. Sometimes finding out exactly what the patient does at work can be helpful. Note particularly any work exposure to dusts, chemicals or disease; for example, mine workers may have the disease silicosis. Checking on hobbies can also be informative (e.g., bird fanciers and lung disease).

SOCIAL HABITS

This is the time when possibly awkward questions about the patients habits should be asked.

Smoking

The patient may claim to be a non-smoker if he or she stopped smoking that morning. Therefore, one must ask if the patient has ever smoked and, if so, how many cigarettes (or cigars or pipes) were smoked a day and for how many years. Cigarette smoking is a risk factor for vascular disease, chronic lung disease and several cancers, and may damage the fetus.

Alcohol

Ask if the patient drinks alcohol. It is useful to ask first what the patient usually drinks (e.g., beer or wine) and then how many glasses a day. It can be useful at this stage to 'adjust up' the patient's estimate (e.g., 'So you drink about 10 beers a day, do you drink any spirits?') giving the patient the chance to modify the original claim without embarrassment.

Remember the maximum safe levels of consumption recommended by the Royal College of Physicians — 21 units a week for men and 17 units a week for women; 1 unit = 10 g of alcohol or about one standard drink (one glass of wine, one middy of standard beer or one nip of spirits).

Certain questions can be helpful in making a diagnosis of alcoholism; these are referred to as the CAGE questions:

1. Have you ever felt you ought to Cut down on your drinking?

2. Have people Annoyed you by criticising your drinking?

3. Have you every felt bad or Guilty about your drinking?

4. Have you every had a drink first thing in the morning to steady your nerves or get rid of a hangover (Eye opener)?

If the patient answers yes to any of these questions, this suggests there may be a serious drinking problem and further inquiry into the history of alcohol use is important.

Analgesics

If the patient has not already volunteered information about the use of analgesics, ask about this. Aspirin and other non-steroidal anti-inflammatory drugs (NSAIDs) but not paracetamol can cause ulcers, gastrointestinal bleeding, asthma and renal impairment.

OVERSEAS TRAVEL

If an infectious disease is a possibility, ask about recent overseas travel, destinations reached, how the patient lived when away and prophylaxis given to protect against diseases such as malaria. People who were born or have lived for long periods overseas may acquire diseases such as tuberculosis.

MARITAL STATUS, SOCIAL SUPPORT AND LIVING CONDITIONS

Inquire about the patient's marital status, including whether there is anyone to help with convalescence. A useful way to start is to ask 'Who is at home with you?' Find out about the health of the spouse or partner and of any children.

SEXUAL AND DRUG ABUSE HISTORY

The sexual history is relevant, particularly if there is a history of urethral discharge, dysuria (burning or pain on urination), vaginal discharge, a genital ulcer or rash, pain on intercourse or anorectal symptoms, or if the acquired immunodeficiency syndrome (AIDS) or hepatitis is suspected.

Approaching this topic is never easy for the doctor or patient. You may wish to preface these questions with a statement such as 'I need to ask you some personal questions because they may be relevant to your current state of health.' It is not the clinician's role to make judgments about a person's life.

Determine the last date of intercourse, number of contacts, homosexual or bisexual partners, and contacts with prostitutes. The type of sexual practice may also be important: for example, oro-anal contact may predispose to colonic infection, and perirectal contact to hepatitis B, C or AIDS, while inserting objects into the rectum may cause trauma.

The use of intravenous drugs has many implications for the patient's health. Ask if an attempt is made to avoid the sharing of needles. This may protect against the injection of viruses but not against bacterial infection from the use of impure substances.

MILY HISTORY

...un in families. For example, ischaemic heart disease in parents who developed this at a young age is a major risk factor for ischaemic heart disease in the offspring. Various malignancies, such as breast and large bowel carcinoma, are more common in certain families. It may be worth asking specifically about a family history of heart disease, stroke, diabetes, tuberculosis, alcoholism, bleeding tendencies or gout. Some diseases are directly inherited (e.g., haemophilia). Ask whether similar illnesses have occurred in other family members but ignore long stories about suspected exotic illnesses in distant cousins.

■ SYSTEMS REVIEW

As well as detailed questioning in the system likely to be diseased, asking about important symptoms and disorders in other systems is essential, otherwise important diseases may be missed. The extent of this review depends on the presenting problem and circumstances. An 18 year old man needing sutures will clearly require less interrogation than a 75 year old with multiple medical problems.

Ask where relevant about key symptoms and common disorders in each major system as described below.

CARDIOVASCULAR SYSTEM

- Have you had any pain or pressure in your chest? (angina).

- Are you short of breath on exertion? (dyspnoea). How much exertion is necessary? How many flights of stairs can you climb before you start to become short of breath?

- Have you ever been woken at night by shortness of breath? (paroxysmal nocturnal dyspnoea).

- Can you lie flat without feeling breathless? (orthopnoea). Have you had swelling of your ankles (peripheral oedema), or varicose veins?

- Have you noticed your heart racing or beating irregularly?
- Do you have pain in your calves on walking? (claudication).
- Do you have cold or blue hands or feet? (peripheral cyanosis).
- Have you ever had rheumatic fever, a heart attack, or high blood pressure?

RESPIRATORY SYSTEM

- Are you short of breath at rest?
- Have you had any cough?
- Do you cough up anything? (productive cough).
- Have you coughed up blood? (haemoptysis).
- Do you snore loudly or fall asleep during the day unexpectedly? (possible obstructive sleep apnoea).
- Do you ever have wheezing when you are short of breath? (bronchospasm).
- Have you had fevers recently?
- Do you have night sweats?
- Have you ever had pneumonia or tuberculosis?
- Have you had a recent chest X-ray?

BREASTS (WOMEN)

- Have you had any bleeding or discharge from your breasts?
- Have you felt any lumps there?
- Have you had a mammogram?

GASTROINTESTINAL SYSTEM

- Have you had a sore tongue or mouth ulcers?

- Are you troubled by indigestion? What do you mean by indigestion?
- Have you been taking antacids or over-the-counter indigestion medicines?
- Have you had pain or discomfort in your belly (tummy)?
- Have you had any bloating or visible swelling of your belly?
- Has your bowel habit changed recently?
- How many bowel motions a week do you usually pass?
- Have you lost control of your bowels or had accidents? (faecal incontinence).
- Have you seen blood in your motions (haematochezia) or vomited blood? (haematemesis).
- Have your bowel motions been black? (melaena).
- Do you take laxatives or enemas?
- Have you had any difficulty swallowing? (dysphagia).
- Has your appetite or weight changed? How has it changed?
- Do you have heartburn?
- Have your eyes or skin ever been yellow? (jaundice).
- Have you noticed dark urine and pale stools?
- Have you ever had hepatitis, peptic ulceration, colitis, or bowel cancer?
- Tell me about your diet recently.

GENITOURINARY SYSTEM

- Do you have burning or pain (dysuria) on passing urine?
- Is your urine stream as good as it used to be?
- Is there a delay before you start to pass urine? (hesitancy).
- Is there dribbling at the end when you pass urine?
- Do you have to get up at night to pass urine? (nocturia).

- Are you passing larger or smaller amounts of urine?
- Have you noticed leaking of urine? (incontinence).
- Has the urine colour changed? Is your urine dark?
- Have you seen blood in the urine? (haematuria).
- Have you any problems with your sex life? Are you impotent?
- Have you noticed any rashes or lumps on your genitals?
- Have you ever had venereal disease? Have you had a penile discharge or skin lesions?
- Have you ever felt lumps in your testes?
- Have you ever had a urinary tract infection or kidney stones?
- Are your periods regular? At what age did you begin to menstruate? (menarche).
- Do you have excessive pain (dysmenorrhoea) or bleeding (menorrhagia) with your periods?
- Do you have bleeding after sex?
- Have you had any miscarriages? (Remember the Gravida number is the number of pregnancies and the Para number is the number of births of babies of over 20 weeks gestation.)
- Have you had high blood pressure or diabetes in pregnancy?

HAEMATOLOGICAL SYSTEM

- Do you bruise easily?
- Have you had bleeding from your gums?
- Have you had fevers, or shivers and shakes (rigors)?
- Do you have difficulty stopping a small cut from bleeding?
- Have you noticed any lumps under your arms, or in your neck or groin?

- Have you ever had blood clots in your legs (venous thrombosis) or in the lungs (pulmonary embolism)?

MUSCULOSKELETAL SYSTEM

- Do you have painful or stiff joints? What joints are affected?
- Are your joints ever hot or red or swollen?
- Have you had muscle pains or cramps?
- Have you had a skin rash recently?
- Do you have any back or neck pain?
- Have your eyes been dry or red?
- Is your mouth often dry?
- Have you been diagnosed as having rheumatoid arthritis or gout?
- Do your fingers ever become painful and go white and blue in the cold? (Raynaud's phenomenon).

ENDOCRINE SYSTEM

- Have you noticed any swelling in your neck? (goitre).
- Do your hands tremble? (tremor).
- Do you prefer hot or cold weather?
- Have you had a thyroid problem or diabetes?
- Have you noticed increased sweating?
- Have you been troubled by fatigue?
- Have you noticed any change in your appearance, hair, skin or voice?
- Have you noticed a change in hat, glove or shoe size? (acromegaly).
- Have you been unusually thirsty lately?

NEUROLOGICAL SYSTEM AND MENTAL STA

- Do you get headaches?
- Have you had memory problems or trouble concentrating?
- Have you had fainting episodes, fits or blackouts?
- Do you have double vision (diplopia) or other trouble seeing or hearing?
- Are you dizzy? Does the world seem to turn around? (vertigo).
- Have you had weakness or numbness or clumsiness in your arms or legs or trouble with balance or walking?
- Have you ever had a stroke or serious head injury?
- Have you had difficulty sleeping?
- Do you feel sad or depressed or have problems with your nerves?
- Have you ever considered suicide?

SKIN

- Have you had itching (pruritus) or a rash?
- Have you noticed moles that have changed?
- Has there been a change in your hair or nails?
- Have you had lumps or frequent infections in the skin?

Is there anything else you would like to talk about?

ACTIVITIES OF DAILY LIVING (ADLs)

For elderly patients and those with a chronic illness, as part of the review of symptoms, some basic screening questions about **functional activity** should be asked. These include ability to bathe,

...et, and eat and dress. There should also be ...e **instrumental activities** of daily living such as ... and cleaning, the use of transport, and manag-...edications.

BEGINNING THE EXAMINATION

EQUIPMENT

A sense of excitement usually accompanies the acquisition of examination tools by the new medical student. This excitement should not lead to the purchase of exotic and expensive equipment. This is not only unnecessary but it also may be unwise to present on the first day with a gold plated stethoscope clearly superior to that of the teaching staff; it leaves very little excuse for not being able to hear soft murmurs.

Most students equip themselves with a number of frequently used items. The most glamorous and indeed most useful (except for the only really vital tool — a pen) is the stethoscope. Many types are available and most work well. It is said that it is what is between the ear-pieces of the stethoscope that really matters. There is some advantage in having a separate tube for each ear. These may be bound in a single outer tube or separated but they should not bounce together and make distracting noises. The stethoscope needs to be robust and easily squashed into different sized pockets. It must also be comfortable when worn in the current fashionable position (e.g., slung over one shoulder). Some newer models do not have a separate bell and diaphragm.

Most other equipment can be obtained on the wards but it is worth acquiring a small pocket ophthalmoscope, a torch and a short patellar hammer. More senior students can usually give advice about the most reliable and inexpensive models available.

GENERAL APPEARANCE

Before the specific examination of the regions or medical systems of the body begins, a general inspection must be made. Make a conscious effort and take the time to consider the patient's appearance, including the face (Table 1.5), hands (Table 1.6) and

TABLE 1.5 Some Important Diagnostic Facies

Acromegalic — prominent chin and supra-orbital ridges

Cushingoid — plethoric and fat

Down syndrome — epicanthic folds, large tongue

Hippocratic (advanced peritonitis) — eyes are sunken, temples collapsed, nose is pinched with crusts on the lips and the forehead is clammy

Marfanoid — thin, high arched palate

Mitral — malar flush (bluish discolouration)

Myopathic — frontal balding, triangular, wasted masseters and thick spectacles or intra-ocular lens implantation (dystrophia myotonica; cataract extraction)

Myxoedematous — puffy, lacking in expression, skin thickening, thinning hair, loss of outer one-third of eyebrows

Pagetic — large cranium

Parkinsonian — expressionless, infrequent blinking

Thyrotoxic — thyroid stare, lid retraction, exopthalmus

Virile facies — acne and facial hair in women

TABLE 1.6 Nail Signs in Systemic Disease

Nail sign	Some causes
Blue nails	Cyanosis, Wilson's disease, ochronosis
Red nails	Polycythaemia (reddish-blue), carbon monoxide poisoning (cherry-red)
Clubbing	Lung cancer, chronic pulmonary suppuration, infective endocarditis, cyanotic congenital heart disease
Splinter haemorrhages	Infective endocarditis, vasculitis
Koilonychia (spoon-shaped nails)	Iron deficiency
Pale nail bed	Anaemia
Onycholysis (separation of nail from nail bed)	Thyrotoxicosis, psoriasis
Leuconychia (white nails)	Hypoalbuminaemia
Nail fold erythema and telangiectasia	Systemic lupus erythematosus

body. Certain facies and body habituses are diagnostic or nearly so. Important relevant signs may be missed unless this is done. For example, the patient with loss of weight may not be identified as having thyrotoxicosis (see Chapter 7) unless the eye signs (e.g., thyroid stare) are noticed.

 FIRST IMPRESSIONS

Is the patient relatively well or very ill?

Specific abnormalities will sometimes be recognised. Look particularly for jaundice (yellow discolouration of the skin and sclerae), cyanosis (blue discolouration of the skin), pallor (suggesting anaemia), or one of the diagnostic facies (Table 1.5).

 VITAL SIGNS

These are indicators of the function of essential parts of the body. They should be assessed in all patients at the time of the initial examination and then as often as necessary.

1. Examine the **radial pulse**. It is usually palpable just medial to the radius with the pulps of the forefinger and middle finger of the examining hand. Estimate or count the rate and note the rhythm (see page 54) (Figure 1.1).

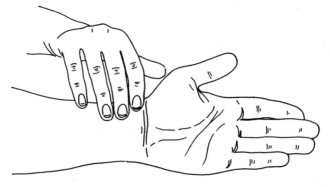

FIGURE 1.1 Taking the radial pulse.

2. Measure the **blood pressure** (Figure 1.2). The usual blood pressure cuff width is 12.5 cm. This is suitable for a normal-sized adult forearm. However, in obese patients with large arms, this cuff will overestimate the blood pressure and therefore a large cuff must be used. A range of smaller sizes is available for children.

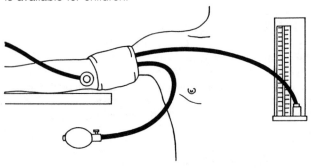

Phase	Korotkoff sounds	
		120 mm Hg systolic
1	A thud	
		110 mm Hg
2	A blowing noise	
		100 mm Hg
3	A softer thud	
		90 mm Hg diastolic (1st)
4	A disappearing blowing noise	
		80mm Hg diastolic (2nd)
5	Nothing	

FIGURE 1.2 Taking the blood pressure.

The cuff is wrapped around the upper arm (which should be supported at the level of the heart) and the bladder centred over the brachial artery. This is found in the antecubital fossa immediately medial to the biceps tendon. For an approximate estimation of the systolic blood pressure, the cuff is fully inflated and then deflated slowly (2 mmHg per second) until the radial pulse returns. Then for a more accurate estimation of the blood pressure, this manoeuvre is repeated with the stethoscope placed over the brachial artery.

Five sounds will be heard as the cuff is slowly released (Figure 1.2). These are called the Korotkoff sounds. The pressure at which a sound is first heard over the artery is the systolic blood pressure (Korotkoff I). As deflation of the cuff continues the sound increases in intensity (K II), then decreases (K III), becomes muffled (K IV) and then disappears (K V). Disappearance (K V) is normally taken to indicate the level of the diastolic pressure.

The systolic blood pressure may normally vary between the arms by up to 10 mmHg; in the legs where it can be taken with a special large cuff, the blood pressure is normally higher than in the arms (this is **not** routine).

During inspiration, the systolic and diastolic blood pressure normally decrease. When this normal reduction in blood pressure with inspiration is exaggerated, it is termed **pulsus paradoxus**. A fall of more than 10 mmHg in arterial pulse pressure on inspiration is abnormal and may occur with constrictive pericarditis, pericardial effusion, or severe asthma.

3. Take the **temperature**. A mercury thermometer is shaken in the traditional way and then placed under the tongue, in the axilla or sometimes in the rectum for 2 minutes and then read. Electronic thermometers which beep in a helpful way when ready have replaced mercury ones in many hospitals. The normal temperature in the mouth is 37 °C and is about 1 °C less in the axilla and about 1 °C more if taken in the rectum.

4. Count the **respiratory rate**. The normal is about 14 breaths a minute. An increased rate may be due to lung disease of almost any type, cardiac failure, metabolic disturbances such as acidosis, or to psychological conditions such as anxiety.

WEIGHT, BODY HABITUS AND POSTURE

Look specifically for obesity, wasting (loss of muscle mass), an unusual facial appearance (Table 1.5) or an abnormal body shape (e.g., the tall thin appearance with long fingers that occurs in Marfan's syndrome).

Weigh the patient. For children the height should also be measured and a weight-height chart consulted to determine the child's growth percentile.

Inspect for limb deformity or missing limbs (these are not always obvious if the patient is huddled under the bed clothes). If the patient walks into the examining room the opportunity to examine gait should not be lost; the full testing of gait is described in Chapter 5.

Assess the state of **hydration**. Severe dehydration is associated with sunken orbits, dry mucous membranes (e.g., tongue), reduced skin elasticity (turgor — an area of skin when pulled away from the body hangs in a wrinkled state for some seconds before falling back) and hypotension (low blood pressure).

Look for **pallor** which may indicate anaemia and for **cyanosis** (see page 25).

THE HANDS AND NAILS

Examination of a system of the body often begins with inspection of the hands and nails. For example the patient with suspected chronic liver disease may have large white lunules in the nails (liver nails) and red palms (palmar erythema). Nail and finger changes may also occur in cardiac and respiratory diseases, endocrine diseases (e.g., acromegaly), arthritis, neurological disease and anaemia (Figure 1.3).

HOW TO EXAMINE A LUMP

Lumps may be present anywhere on the surface of the body. They are usually readily examined and one must have an approach that helps work out the cause.

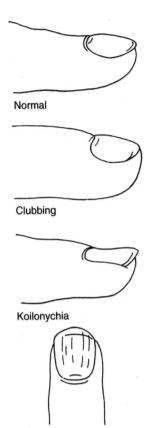

Normal

Clubbing

Koilonychia

Splinter haemorrhages

Pitting

Clubbing occurs in specific diseases:

Heart

infectious endocarditis

cyanotic congenital heart disease

Lungs

carcinoma of the bronchus

chronic infection

– *abscess*

– *bronchiectasis*

– *empyema*
(not chronic bronchitis)

Liver – *cirrhosis*

Congenital

Koilonychia can occur in *iron deficiency anaemia*

Splinter haemorrhages occur in *infectious endocarditis* but are more common in people doing manual work

Pitting occurs in *psoriasis* and *psoriatic arthritis*

FIGURE 1.3   Nail changes.

First, look at and feel the lump to work out its anatomical **site** on the body and its **size**, **shape** and **consistency** (soft or hard). Note if it is **tender** or not.

Next, work out in what tissue layer the lump is situated. If it is in the **skin** (e.g., sebaceous cyst, epidermoid cyst, papilloma), it should move when the skin is moved, but if it is in the **subcutaneous tissue** (e.g., neurofibroma, lipoma), the skin can be moved over the lump. If it is in the **muscle** or **tendon** (e.g., tumour), then contraction of the muscle or tendon will limit the lump's mobility, and mobility is greater in the transverse than the longitudinal axis. If it is in a **nerve**, pressing on the lump may result in pins and needles being felt in the distribution of the nerve and the lump cannot be moved in the longitudinal axis but can be moved in the transverse axis. If it is in **bone**, the lump will be immobile.

Find out if the lump is **fluctuant** (i.e., contains fluid; Figure 1.4). Place one forefinger (the 'watch' finger) halfway between the centre and periphery of the lump. The forefinger from the other hand (the 'displacing' finger) is placed diagonally opposite the first at an

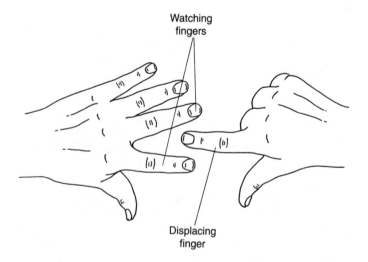

Watching
fingers

Displacing
finger

FIGURE 1.4   Testing a lump for fluctuation.

equal distance from the centre of the lump. Press with the displacing finger and keep the watching finger still. If the lump contains fluid, the watching finger will be displaced in **both** axes of the lump (i.e., fluctuation is present). Place a small torch behind the lump to determine if it can be **transilluminated**.

Note any associated signs of **inflammation** (i.e., redness, swelling, heat and tenderness).

Look for similar lumps elsewhere, (e.g., multiple subcutaneous swellings from neurofibromas or lipomas).

If an inflammatory or neoplastic lump is suspected, remember always to examine the regional lymphatic field, and the other lymph node groups as explained in Chapter 4.

REMEMBER TO DESCRIBE

Site	Colour	Temperature
Size	Contour	Tenderness
Shape	Consistency	Tethering

PREPARING THE PATIENT FOR EXAMINATION

The clinician should try to ensure the patient is comfortable and positioned so as to assist the examination. At each stage the patient should be informed about what is going to happen.

The patient must be undressed so that the parts to be examined are accessible. Modesty requires that a woman's breasts be covered temporarily with a gown or sheet while other parts of the body are being examined. Men and women should both have the groin covered, for example during the examination of the legs. However, important physical signs will be missed in some patients if excessive attention is paid to modesty. The position of the patient in bed or elsewhere should depend on what is to be examined. For example, a patient's abdomen is best examined if he or she lies completely flat so that the abdominal muscles are relaxed. Traditionally, the doctor examines from the right side of the bed.

Every effort should be made to ensure that the examination is not uncomfortable or embarrassing for the patient. The curtains should be drawn around the bed and members of the clinician's entourage should be introduced. The clinician should attempt to warm the examining hands and stethoscope before they are applied to the patient's skin.

TAKING A GOOD HISTORY — HINTS

1. **Allow patients to tell the story in their own words at the beginning. Establish rapport and listen with enthusiasm. Then ask specific questions to fill in the gaps. The patient should not have the impression that the interview is being hurried (except in an emergency).**

2. **Concentrate on the history of the presenting illness. This must be documented sequentially and in the greatest detail.**

3. **Don't forget to explore psychological issues where they may be relevant.**

4. **Begin formulating the differential diagnosis based on the historical information given. Many diagnoses can be identified based on a good history.**

5. **The relevant symptoms obtained on the systems review should be incorporated into the history of the presenting illness.**

6. **Past history, social history and family history are often highly relevant to the presenting illness.**

7. **Systematic questions about potential risk factors for various diseases may assist in establishing the diagnosis (e.g., smoking and coronary artery disease).**

8. **Constant practice is needed if one is to become a proficient history taker.**

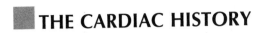

The heart

THE CARDIAC HISTORY

PRESENTING SYMPTOMS (Table 2.1)

Chest Pain

The cause of chest pain is likely to be clearer when questions about the quality, duration, location, precipitating and aggravating factors, means of relief and accompanying symptoms have been answered. **Typical ischaemic chest pain** is due to inadequate blood supply to the myocardium. It is often described as a central or retrosternal (behind the sternum) discomfort rather than a pain. There is frequently a tight or heavy sensation which may radiate to the left arm or to the jaw. It tends to occur on exertion and may be predictable at certain levels of activity. Relief is usually rapid with rest or sub-lingual (under the tongue) nitrate drugs. Prolonged ischaemic type pain or discomfort which comes on at rest is more suggestive of myocardial infarction than angina. The pain of infarction is more likely to be associated with sweating than that of angina.

Unless a careful history is taken, and the association with exertion noted, the clinician and the patient may incorrectly assume lower chest discomfort is due to indigestion rather than to angina.

Consult Table 2.2 for other causes of chest pain.

Dyspnoea

Shortness of breath may be due to cardiac disease. In this case it is often associated with **orthopnoea** (breathlessness that is worse when the patient lies flat) and **paroxysmal nocturnal dyspnoea** (breathlessness that wakes the patient from sleep — typically the patient gets up and walks to the window to breath in fresh air and it takes several minutes for relief to occur).

TABLE 2.1 Cardiovascular History

Major Symptoms
Chest pain or heaviness
Dyspnoea: exertional (note degree of exercise
  necessary), orthopnoea, paroxysmal nocturnal
  dyspnoea
Ankle swelling
Palpitations
Syncope
Intermittent claudication
Fatigue

Past History
Rheumatic fever, chorea, recent (<3 months) dental
  work, thyroid disease
Prior medical examination revealing heart disease
  (e.g., military, school, insurance)
Drugs

Social History
Tobacco and alcohol use
Occupation

Family History
Myocardial infarcts, cardiomyopathy, congenital heart
  disease, mitral valve prolapse, Marfan's syndrome

Coronary Artery Disease Risk Factors
Hyperlipidaemia
Hypertension
Smoking
Family history of coronary artery disease
Diabetes mellitus
Obesity and physical inactivity
Male sex and advanced age

TABLE 2.2 Causes of Chest Pain

Cardiac pain	Myocardial ischaemia or infarction
Vascular pain	Aortic dissection Aortic aneurysm
Pleuropericardial pain	Pericarditis Infective pleurisy Pneumothorax Pneumonia Autoimmune disease Mesothelioma Metastatic tumour
Chest wall pain	Persistent cough Muscular strains Intercostal myositis Thoracic herpes zoster Coxsackie B infection Thoracic nerve compression or infiltration Rib fracture Rib tumour, primary or metastatic Tietze's syndrome
Gastrointestinal pain	Gastroesophageal reflux (common) Oesophageal spasm (uncommon)
Airway pain	Tracheitis Central bronchial carcinoma Inhaled foreign body

TABLE 2.2 Continued

Mediastinal pain	Mediastinitis
	Sarcoid adenopathy
	Lymphoma

Cardiac dyspnoea can be difficult to distinguish from that due to other causes, for example, lung disease. A history of diseases that can cause cardiac failure may help (e.g., previous myocardial infarction, hypertension or valvular heart disease).

Ankle Swelling

Peripheral oedema may be a symptom (and sign) of cardiac failure but there are other more common causes of ankle swelling (e.g., varicose veins, vasodilating drugs).

Palpitations

This is usually taken to mean an unexpected awareness of the heartbeat. Try to find out precisely what it is the patient is aware of. Ask about the perceived heart rate, suddenness of onset and offset and the regularity or irregularity of the heartbeat. It may help to get the patient to tap out the rhythm of the heartbeat with a finger.

Syncope and Dizziness

Syncope is a transient loss of consciousness resulting from cerebral anoxia.

One must establish whether the patient actually loses consciousness and under what circumstances the syncope occurred (e.g., postural syncope — occurs on standing; micturition syncope — occurs when the patient is passing urine; tussive — cough syncope; or vasovagal syncope with sudden emotional stress). The differential diagnosis includes epilepsy, where there may be associated tonic and clonic jerks (rhythmical contraction and relaxation of muscle groups). Aortic stenosis (page 49) or hypertrophic cardiomyopathy (page 53) may be associated with syncope that occurs on exertion. The cause is uncertain but is probably related to inappropriate vasodilatation and hypotension from stimulation of ventricular mechanoreceptors.

Dizziness which occurs even when the patient is lying down or which is made worse by movements of the head is more likely to be of neurological or middle ear origin (page 129). The subjective sensation that the world is turning around suggests **vertigo**, which can be due to vestibular abnormalities (e.g., labyrinthitis).

Intermittent Claudication

A history of claudication (pain in the calves when walking a predictable distance) suggests peripheral vascular disease causing an inadequate blood supply to the affected muscles (page 63).

Fatigue

Fatigue is a common symptom of cardiac failure but there are many other causes of this symptom including depression and hypothyroidism.

RISK FACTORS FOR CORONARY ARTERY AND VALVULAR HEART DISEASE

Previous episodes of ischaemic heart disease, hypercholesterolaemia, smoking, hypertension, a family history of coronary artery disease (first degree relatives — siblings or parents — affected before the age of 60), diabetes mellitus, male sex and advancing age are important risk factors for ischaemic heart disease.

A history of rheumatic fever places patients at risk for rheumatic valvular heart disease.

TREATMENT

This includes current and past drug treatment, the cardiac surgical history and any history of coronary artery angioplasty or balloon valvuloplasty.

SOCIAL AND OCCUPATIONAL HISTORY

This is relevant for any patient with a chronic illness and must be recorded. The availability of family and financial support is important for any patient with a serious illness and may affect such issues as how soon the patient can go home.

Many cardiac conditions affect a patient's ability to work. Heavy physical work may not be possible following an infarct or valve surgery. Certain specific occupations (e.g., commercial flying or vehicle driving) are precluded in patients with certain heart diseases if there is an increased risk of syncope or sudden death.

EXAMINING THE HEART

The mechanical function of the heart results in movement that is often palpable and sometimes visible on the part of the chest that lies in front of it — the praecordium. The passage of blood through the heart and its valves and on into the great vessels of the body produces many interesting and amusing sounds and causes pulsation in arteries and movement in veins in remote parts of the body. Signs of cardiac disease may be found by examining the praecordium and the many accessible arteries and veins of the body.

Examination of the cardiovascular system usually begins with the peripheral signs of heart and vascular disease (such as the pulse, blood pressure and jugular venous pressure). These are described later in this chapter.

POSITIONING THE PATIENT

It is important to begin with the patient lying in bed with enough pillows to support him or her at 45° (Figure 2.1). In this position the chest is easily accessible and this is the usual position in which the jugular venous pressure is assessed (see page 60).

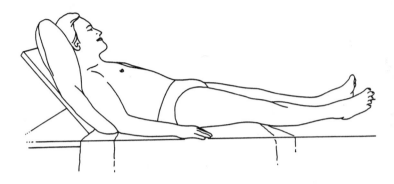

FIGURE 2.1   Patient at 45° angle.

THE PRAECORDIUM

Inspection

You will be **looking** (i) at the chest wall for scars and lumps; and (ii) for the apex beat (visible contraction of the left ventricle during systole).

Inspect first for **scars**. Previous cardiac operations will have left scars on the chest wall. Coronary artery and valve surgery are usually performed through a median sternotomy incision and a scar will be visible extending from just below the supra-sternal notch to the xiphisternum.

Another surgical 'abnormality' is a **pacemaker box**. These are usually under the right or left pectoral muscle, are easily palpable and obviously metallic.

The **apex beat** (Figure 2.2) may be visible as a flickering movement of a small area (about the size of a 20 cent or 50p piece) of the skin of the chest wall between two ribs. It is caused by the twisting or wringing movement that occurs with ventricular systole (contraction). Its normal position is in the fifth left intercostal space 1 cm medial to the midclavicular line (Figure 2.2).

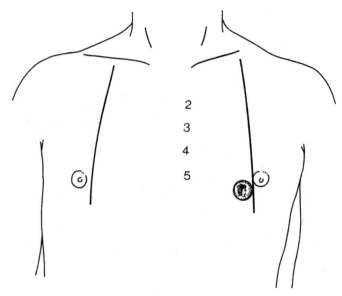

FIGURE 2.2   The apex beat.

Palpation

You will be trying to **feel** for:

1. the apex beat;
2. thrills (palpable murmurs); and
3. other impulses.

Count down the number of interspaces to where the apex beat is palpable (Figure 2.2). The first palpable rib interspace is the second. The position of the apex beat is defined as the most lateral and inferior point at which the palpating fingers are raised with each systole. An apex beat displaced laterally or inferiorly or both usually indicates enlargement of the heart, but may occasionally be due to chest wall deformity, or pleural or pulmonary disease.

The normal apex beat gently lifts the palpating fingers. Try to decide if the apex beat is normal or one of the five types of abnormal apex beat.

1. The **dyskinetic** apex beat feels uncoordinated and large. It is usually due to left ventricular dysfunction (for example, anterior myocardial infarction).

2. The **volume loaded** (hyperkinetic or diastolic overloaded) apex beat is a coordinated impulse felt over a larger area than normal in the praecordium and is usually the result of left ventricular dilatation, for example, due to aortic regurgitation.

3. The **pressure loaded** (hyperdynamic or systolic overloaded) apex beat is a forceful and sustained impulse. This occurs with aortic stenosis or hypertension.

4. The **double impulse** apex beat, where two distinct impulses are felt with each systole, is characteristic of hypertrophic cardiomyopathy (an inherited condition involving hypertrophy of the interventricular cardiac septum).

5. The **tapping apex** beat will be felt where the first heart sound is actually palpable (heart sounds are not palpable in health) and usually indicates mitral stenosis.

In some cases the apex beat may not be palpable. This is most often due to lack of practice, a thick chest wall, emphysema, pericardial effusion, shock (or death) and very rarely to dextrocardia (where there is inversion of the heart and great vessels). The apex beat will be palpable to the right of the sternum in many cases of dextrocardia.

Turbulent blood flow, which is what causes cardiac murmurs on auscultation, may sometimes be palpable. These palpable murmurs are called **thrills**. The praecordium should be systematically palpated for thrills with the flat of the hand (palm side), first over the apex and left sternal edge, and then over the base of the heart (this is the upper part of the chest and includes the aortic and pulmonary areas; Figure 2.3).

Apical thrills can be more easily felt with the patient rolled over to the left side (the left lateral position) as this brings the apex closer to the chest wall. Thrills may also be palpable over the **base of the heart**. These may be maximum over the pulmonary or aortic

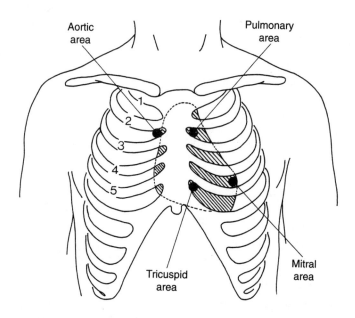

FIGURE 2.3 Areas of auscultation.

areas, depending on the underlying cause and are best felt with the patient sitting up leaning forward and in full expiration. In this position the base of the heart is moved closer to the chest wall. A thrill which coincides in time with the apex beat is called a **systolic thrill**; one which does not coincide with the apex beat is called a **diastolic thrill**.

The presence of a thrill usually means there is a significant abnormality of the heart and that the associated murmur is not an **innocent** (normal variation) murmur.

Feel also for a **parasternal impulse**. The heel of the hand is rested just to the left of the sternum with the fingers lifted slightly off the chest. In cases of right ventricular enlargement or severe left atrial enlargement, where the right ventricle is pushed anteriorly, the heel of the hand is lifted off the chest wall with each systole.

Palpation with the fingers over the pulmonary area (second left intercostal space) may reveal the palpable tap of pulmonary valve closure (P2) in cases of pulmonary hypertension.

Auscultation

You will be **listening** in each area of the heart for:

1. the heart sounds (first and second);

2. extra heart sounds (third and fourth);

3. additional sounds (e.g., snaps, clicks or prosthetic heart sounds);

4. murmurs (which you will need to time, determine the area of greatest intensity, assess loudness and pitch; and, if indicated, perform dynamic manoeuvres for); and

5. rubs.

Auscultation of the heart begins in the mitral area (Figure 2.3) with the bell of the stethoscope. This better amplifies low pitched sounds such as the murmur of mitral stenosis. It must be applied lightly to the chest wall. Next listen in the mitral area with the diaphragm of the stethoscope, which best reproduces higher pitched sounds, such as the systolic murmur of mitral regurgitation. Then place the stethoscope in the tricuspid area (fifth left intercostal space) and listen. Next inch up the left sternal edge to the pulmonary (second left intercostal space) and aortic (second right intercostal space) areas, listening carefully in each position with the diaphragm (Figure 2.4).

Auscultation of the normal heart reveals two sounds called, not surprisingly, the first and second heart sounds.

The **first heart sound (S1)** has two components: mitral and tricuspid valve closure. Mitral closure occurs slightly before tricuspid, but usually only one sound is audible. The first heart sound indicates the beginning of ventricular contraction (systole — ventricular relaxation is called diastole).

The **second heart sound (S2)** at the apex is generally softer, shorter and higher pitched than the first (Figure 2.5). It marks the end of systole and is made up of sounds from aortic and pulmonary valve closures. In normal cases, because of lower pressure in

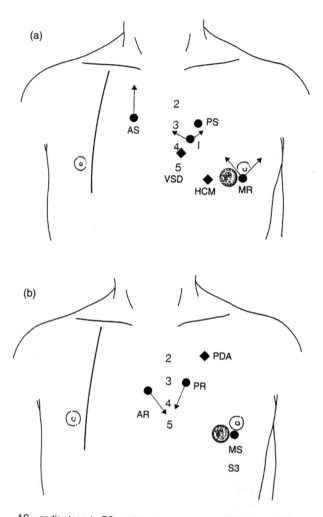

AS = aortic stenosis; PS = pulmonary stenosis; MR = mitral regurgitation;
VSD = ventricular septal defect; HCM = hypertrophic cardiomyopathy;
PDA = patent ductus arteriosus; PR = pulmonary regurgitation;
AR = aortic regurgitation; MS = mitral stenosis; S3 = third heart sound.

FIGURE 2.4 Radiation and sites of maximum intensity
of murmurs.

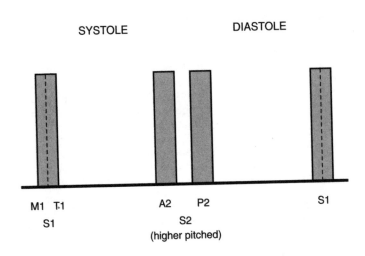

SYSTOLE   DIASTOLE

M1 T1   A2   P2   S1
S1   S2
                    (higher pitched)

S1 = first heart sound; S2 = second heart sound;
M1 = mitral component of S1; T1 = tricuspid component of S1;
A2 = aortic component of S2; P2 = pulmonary component of S2.

FIGURE 2.5   Normal heart sounds.

the pulmonary circulation compared with the aorta, closure of the pulmonary valve is later than that of the aortic valve. These components are usually sufficiently separated in time so that **splitting** of the second heart sound is audible and is best appreciated in the pulmonary area and along the left sternal edge. Pulmonary valve closure is further delayed with inspiration because of increased venous return to the right ventricle, and thus splitting of the second heart sound is wider on inspiration. The second heart sound marks the beginning of diastole, which is usually longer than systole.

It can be difficult to decide which heart sound is which. Palpation of the carotid pulsation in the neck (page 59) will indicate the timing of systole and enable the heart sounds to be more easily distinguished.

Abnormalities of the Heart Sounds

ALTERATIONS IN INTENSITY

The first heart sound (S1) is loud when the mitral or tricuspid valve cusps remain widely open at the end of diastole and shut forcefully with the onset of ventricular systole. This occurs in mitral stenosis.

Soft first heart sounds can be due to failure of the leaflets to coapt normally (as in mitral regurgitation).

The second heart sound (S2) may have a **loud** aortic component (A2) in patients with systemic hypertension. The pulmonary component of the second heart sound (P2) is loud in pulmonary hypertension, where the valve closure is forceful because of the high pulmonary pressure.

A **soft** A2 will be found when the aortic valve is calcified and leaflet movement is reduced, and in aortic regurgitation when the leaflets cannot coapt.

SPLITTING (Figure 2.6)

Splitting of the first heart sound is usually not detectable clinically; however, when it occurs it is most often due to complete right bundle branch block.

Increased normal splitting (wider on inspiration) of the second heart sound occurs when there is any delay in right ventricular emptying as in right bundle branch block (delayed right ventricular depolarisation) or pulmonary stenosis (delayed right ventricular ejection).

In the case of **fixed splitting** the normal respiratory variation is absent and splitting tends to be wide. This is caused by an atrial septal defect where equalisation of volume loads between the two atria occurs through the defect.

EXTRA HEART SOUNDS

The **third heart sound (S3)** is a low pitched mid-diastolic sound that is best appreciated by listening for the characteristic triple cadence of the cardiac rhythm. It has been likened to the galloping of a horse and is often called a gallop rhythm.

A **left ventricular S3** is louder at the apex than at the left sternal edge, and is louder on expiration. It can be physiological in pregnancy. Otherwise, it is an important sign of left ventricular failure, (Table 2.6) but may also occur in aortic regurgitation (page 51) or mitral regurgitation (page 49).

The **fourth heart sound (S4)** is a late diastolic sound slightly more high pitched than the S3. Again, this is responsible for the impression of a triple (gallop) rhythm. It is never physiological and is most often due to systemic hypertension (page 57).

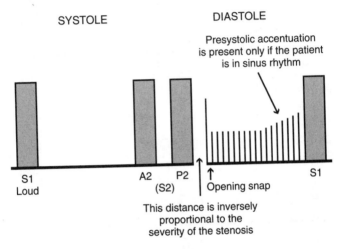

Mitral stenosis (MS) (at the apex).

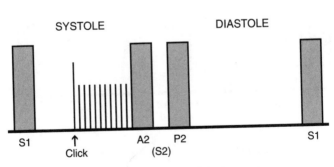

Mitral valve prolapse (MVP) (at the apex).

FIGURE 2.6 Heart sounds, clicks, snaps and splitting.

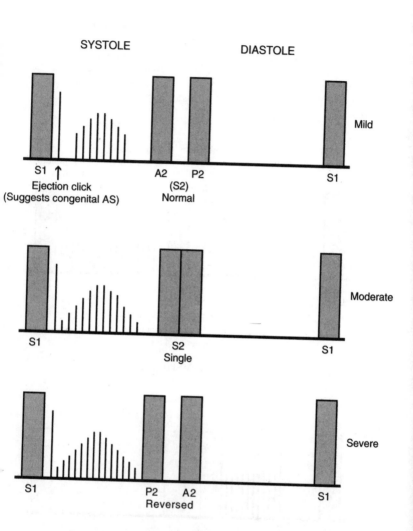

Aortic stenosis (AS) (at the aortic area).

FIGURE 2.6 Continued

ADDITIONAL SOUNDS

An **opening snap** is a high pitched sound which occurs in mitral stenosis at a variable distance after S2 (Figure 2.6). It is due to the sudden opening of the mitral valve and is followed by the diastolic murmur of mitral stenosis. It is best heard at the lower left sternal edge with the diaphragm of the stethoscope. Use of the term *opening snap* implies the diagnosis of mitral (or the very uncommon tricuspid) stenosis.

A **systolic ejection click** is an early systolic high pitched sound heard over the aortic or pulmonary area which may occur in cases of congenital aortic or pulmonary stenosis where the valve remains mobile; it is followed by the systolic ejection murmur of aortic or pulmonary stenosis.

A **non-ejection systolic click** is a high pitched sound heard during systole and is best appreciated at the mitral area. It is a common finding. It may be followed by a systolic murmur. The click may be due to prolapse of one or both redundant mitral valve leaflets during systole.

Mechanical **prosthetic heart valves** produce characteristic crisp metallic sounds.

Murmurs of the Heart

The correct diagnosis of a murmur depends on the synthesis of findings made at the praecordium (apex beat, thrills etc.), the noise itself and peripheral signs (page 55).

TIMING (Table 2.3)

Systolic murmurs (which occur during ventricular systole) may be pansystolic, ejection systolic or late systolic.

The **pansystolic murmur** extends throughout systole beginning with the first heart sound then going right up to the second heart sound. Causes of pansystolic murmurs include some types of mitral regurgitation (Figure 2.4), tricuspid regurgitation and ventricular septal defect.

An **ejection (mid) systolic** murmur does not begin right at the first heart sound; its intensity is greatest in midsystole or later, and wanes again late in systole. This is described as a crescendo-decrescendo murmur. These murmurs are usually caused by turbulent flow through the aortic or pulmonary valve orifices or by

TABLE 2.3 Cardiac Murmurs

Timing	Lesion	Maximum intensity
Pansystolic	Mitral regurgitation	Apex
	Tricuspid regurgitation	LLSE (Lower left sternal edge)
	Ventricular septal defect	
Midsystolic	Aortic stenosis	Base (aortic area)
	Pulmonary stenosis	Base (pulmonary area)
	Hypertrophic cardiomyopathy	LLSE
	Pulmonary flow murmur of an atrial septal defect	(Pulmonary area)
Late systolic	Mitral valve prolapse	Apex
	Papillary muscle dysfunction (due usually to ischaemia or hypertrophic cardiomyopathy)	Apex
Early diastolic	Aortic regurgitation	LLSE
	Pulmonary regurgitation	LSE (Left sternal edge)
Mid-diastolic	Mitral stenosis	Apex
	Tricuspid stenosis	RLSE (Right lower sternal edge)
	Atrial myxoma	Apex

greatly increased flow through a normal sized orifice or outflow tract.

If a murmur is **late systolic**, one is able to distinguish a gap between the first heart sound and the murmur which then continues right up to the second heart sound. This is typical of mitral valve prolapse or papillary muscle dysfunction where mitral regurgitation begins in midsystole.

Diastolic murmurs occur during ventricular diastole. The **early diastolic murmur** begins immediately with the second heart sound and has a decrescendo quality (it is loudest at the beginning and extends for a variable distance into diastole). These early diastolic murmurs are typically high pitched and are due to regurgitation through a leaking aortic or pulmonary valve.

Mid-diastolic murmurs begin later in diastole and may be short or extend right up to the first heart sound. They have a much lower pitched quality than early diastolic murmurs. They are due to impaired flow during ventricular filling and can be caused by mitral stenosis where the valve is narrowed.

Presystolic murmurs may be heard when atrial systole increases blood flow across the valve just before the first heart sound. They are an extension of the mid-diastolic murmurs of mitral stenosis and tricuspid stenosis, and are absent in patients who are in atrial fibrillation (because atrial systole is lost).

Continuous murmurs extend throughout systole and diastole. They are produced when a communication exists between two parts of the circulation with a permanent pressure gradient so that blood flow occurs continuously (e.g., patent [persistent] ductus arteriosus). They should be distinguished from combined systolic and diastolic murmurs (due, for example, to aortic stenosis and aortic regurgitation).

A **pericardial friction rub** is a superficial scratching sound; there may be up to three distinct components occurring at any time during the cardiac cycle. They are not confined to systole or diastole. A rub is caused by movement of inflamed pericardial surfaces. The sound can vary with respiration and posture; it is often louder when the patient is sitting up and breathing out. It tends to come and go.

AREA OF GREATEST INTENSITY

Unfortunately the place on the praecordium where a murmur is loudest is not a very reliable guide to its origin. For example, the murmur of mitral regurgitation, although clearly audible at the apex, may be heard widely over the praecordium and even right up into the aortic area or over the back. Conduction of an ejection systolic murmur up into the carotid arteries, however, suggests that this arises from the aortic valve. The murmur of a ventricular septal defect is loudest in the right parasternal area and is not well heard at the base of the heart or at the apex. This helps distinguish it from the murmurs of aortic stenosis and mitral regurgitation, respectively.

LOUDNESS AND PITCH

The loudness of the murmur is often **not** helpful in deciding the severity of the valve lesion. Harshness is perhaps a better guide. Changes in the loudness, however, are very important. Murmurs are usually graded according to loudness. Cardiologists most often use a classification with six grades.

Grade 1/6: very soft and only audible in ideal listening conditions

Grade 2/6: soft, but can be detected almost immediately by an experienced auscultator

Grade 3/6: moderate; there is no thrill

Grade 4/6: loud; thrill just palpable

Grade 5/6: very loud; thrill easily palpable

Grade 6/6: very, very loud (and very uncommon); it can be heard even without placing the stethoscope on the chest

DYNAMIC MANOEUVRES

Respiration: Listen to the murmur as the patient breathes deeply in and out. Murmurs that arise on the right side of the heart tend to be louder during inspiration as this increases venous return and therefore blood flow to the right side of the heart.

The **Valsalva manoeuvre:** this is a forceful expiration against a closed glottis. One should ask the patient to breath in, hold his or her nose with the fingers, close the mouth, breathe out hard and completely so as to pop the eardrums, and hold this for as long as

TABLE 2.4 Dynamic Manoeuvres and Systolic Cardiac Murmurs

Manoeuvre	Lesion			
	Hypertrophic cardiomyopathy	**Mitral valve prolapse**	**Aortic stenosis**	**Mitral regurgitation**
Valsalva strain phase (decreases preload)	Louder	Longer	Softer	Softer
Squatting or leg raise (increases preload)	Softer	Shorter	Louder	Louder
Hand grip (increases afterload)	Softer	Shorter	Softer	Louder

possible. Listen over the left sternal edge during this manoeuvre for changes in the systolic murmur of hypertrophic cardiomyopathy, and over the apex for changes when mitral valve prolapse is suspected. See Table 2.4.

Exercise: if mitral stenosis is suspected but the diastolic murmur is difficult to hear, it is helpful to exercise the patient by getting him or her to sit up and down a number of times. Get the patient then to lie quickly on the left side and listen at the apex with the bell.

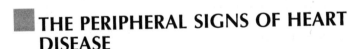

THE PERIPHERAL SIGNS OF HEART DISEASE

GENERAL APPEARANCE

Note the general state of health. Look to see if the patient has rapid and laboured respiration, suggesting dyspnoea which is both a symptom and a sign. Dyspnoea may be present as the patient undresses or even at rest.

Look for cachexia; that is, severe loss of weight and muscle wasting. This is commonly caused by malignant disease, but severe cardiac failure may also produce this appearance (cardiac cachexia).

THE HANDS

Pick up the right hand, then the left. Look for **peripheral cyanosis** which is blue discolouration of the fingers, toes and other peripheral parts of the body. Look at the nails from the side for **clubbing** (Figure 1.3). This is an increase in the soft tissue of the distal part of the fingers or toes, and occurs in cyanotic congenital heart disease (Table 1.6).

Before leaving the nails, look for **splinter haemorrhages** in the nail beds. These are linear haemorrhages lying parallel to the long axis of the nail. They are most often due to trauma, particularly in manual workers. However, an important cause is infective endocarditis which is a bacterial (or less commonly a fungal) infection of the heart valves or part of the endocardium.

Tendon xanthomata are yellow or orange deposits of lipid in the tendons including those of the hand and arm. They occur in hyperlipidaemia.

THE ARTERIAL PULSE (Table 2.5)

The following observations should be made at the radial pulse (page 25): (i) **rate** of pulse; (ii) **rhythm**; and (iii) presence or absence of delay of the femoral pulse compared with the radial pulse (**radiofemoral delay**).

Rate of Pulse

The pulse rate can be counted over 30 seconds and multiplied by two. The normal resting heart rate in adults is between 60 and 100 beats per minute. Bradycardia is defined as a heart rate less than 60 beats per minute. Tachycardia is defined as a heart rate over 100 beats per minute.

TABLE 2.5 Arterial Pulse Character

Type of pulse	Cause(s)
Anacrotic Small volume, slow uptake, notched wave on upstroke	Aortic stenosis
Plateau Slow upstroke	Aortic stenosis
Bisferiens Anacrotic and collapsing	Aortic stenosis *and* regurgitation
Collapsing	Aortic regurgitation Hyperdynamic circulation Patent ductus arteriosus Peripheral arteriovenous fistula Arteriosclerotic aorta (elderly patients in particular)
Small volume	Aortic stenosis Pericardial effusion
Alternans Alternating strong and weak beats	Severe left ventricular failure
Jerky	Hypertrophic cardiomyopathy

TABLE 2.5 Continued

Type of pulse	Cause(s)	
Pulsus paradoxus	Tamponade or severe asthma	
Presystolic	Mitral stenosis	Apex
	Tricuspid stenosis	RLSE
	Atrial myxoma	Apex
Continuous	Patent ductus arteriosus	Below left clavicle
	Arteriovenous fistula (coronary artery, pulmonary, systemic)	LSE
	Aorto-pulmonary connection	LSE
	Venous hum (usually best heard over right supraclavicular fossa and abolished by ipsilateral internal jugular vein compression)	
	Rupture of sinus of Valsalva into right ventricle or atrium 'Mammary souffle' (in late pregnancy or early postpartum period)	LSE

NB: The combined murmurs of aortic stenosis and aortic regurgitation, or mitral stenosis and mitral regurgitation, may sound as if they fill the entire cardiac cycle, but are not continuous murmurs by definition.

Rhythm

The rhythm of the pulse can be regular or irregular. An irregular rhythm can be completely irregular with no pattern; this is usually due to atrial fibrillation which occurs when coordinated contraction of the atria is lost and the ventricles beat irregularly and usually fast. The pulse rate is then usually rapid (greater than 120 beats per minute) unless the patient is being treated with drugs to slow it down. This type of pulse can occasionally be caused by frequent, irregularly occurring supraventricular or ventricular ectopic beats.

An irregular rhythm can also be regularly irregular. For example, in **sinus arrhythmia** the pulse rate increases with each inspiration and decreases with each expiration. This is not abnormal.

Character and Volume

The character and volume of the pulse are better assessed from palpation of the brachial or carotid arteries. However the collapsing (bounding) pulse of aortic regurgitation may be readily apparent at the wrist.

THE BLOOD PRESSURE

The systolic blood pressure (see page 26) is the peak pressure that occurs in the artery following ventricular systole and the diastolic blood pressure is the level to which the arterial blood pressure falls during ventricular diastole.

High Blood Pressure

This is difficult to define. The most helpful definition of hypertension is based on an estimation of the level associated with an increased risk of vascular disease. In this case, recordings above 145mmHg systolic or 90mmHg diastolic are considered abnormal; such levels may occur in up to 20% of the adult population.

Postural Blood Pressure

The blood pressure should routinely be taken with the patient lying and standing. A fall in blood pressure of more than 15mmHg in systolic blood pressure or 10mmHg in diastolic blood pressure on standing is abnormal and is called postural hypotension. It may not be associated with symptoms.

CHANGES WITH RESPIRATION; PULSUS PARADOXUS

A fall in systolic blood pressure of up to 15mmHg occurs normally during inspiration. Exaggeration of this response — a fall of more than 15mmHg is an important sign of pericardial tamponade (rapid accumulation of fluid in the pericardial space) or severe asthma. It is detected by lowering the cuff pressure slowly from a level above the systolic pressure. The expiratory systolic blood pressure will be detected when Korotkoff I sounds (page 27) are heard intermittently. As the cuff pressure is lowered there will be a point when Korotkoff I sounds are heard throughout the respiratory cycle. The difference between these two readings gives the level of pulsus paradoxus.

THE FACE

Xanthelasma are intracutaneous yellow cholesterol deposits around the eyes and are relatively common. These may be a normal variant or may indicate hyperlipidaemia.

In the mouth, use a torch to see if there is a **high arched palate**. This occurs in Marfan's syndrome, a condition which is associated with congenital heart disease, including aortic regurgitation secondary to aortic dilatation, and also mitral regurgitation due to mitral valve prolapse. Look for **diseased teeth** as they can be a source of organisms responsible for infective endocarditis. Look at the tongue and lips for **central cyanosis** which is cyanosis of parts of the body not subject to reduced blood supply in the cold.

THE NECK

Useful information about cardiac function is available in most necks. Arterial (carotid) and venous (jugular) pulsations should be examined.

1. Carotid Arteries

The carotid pulse can be felt medial to the sternomastoid muscle by applying slight posterior and medial pressure with the middle and forefingers (Figure 2.7). Evaluation of the amplitude, shape and volume of the pulse is used to help in the diagnosis of various underlying cardiac diseases and in assessing their severity. Important carotid abnormalities are described in Table 2.3.

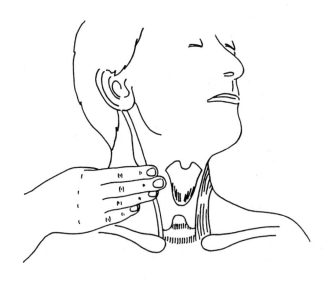

FIGURE 2.7 Feeling the carotid pulse.

2. Jugular Venous Pressure (JVP)

The internal jugular vein runs a direct course to the right atrium (Figure 2.8). By convention, the sternal angle is taken as the zero point and the maximum height of pulsations in the internal jugular vein, which are visible above this level when the patient is at 45°, can be measured in centimetres.

The jugular venous pulsation can be distinguished from the arterial pulse because: (i) it is visible but not palpable; (ii) it has a complex wave form, usually seen to flicker twice with each cardiac cycle (if the patient is in sinus rhythm); (iii) it moves on respiration — normally the JVP decreases on inspiration; and (iv) it is at first obliterated and then filled from above when light pressure is applied at the base of the neck.

The JVP must be assessed for **height** and **character**.

When the JVP is more than 3 cm above the zero point, the right heart filling pressure is raised. This is a sign of right ventricular failure or of volume overload.

There are two positive waves in the normal JVP. The first is called the **a wave** and coincides with right atrial systole. It is due to atrial contraction. The a wave also coincides with the first heart sound and precedes the carotid pulsation. The second impulse is called the **v wave** and is due to atrial filling, in the period when the tricuspid valve remains closed during ventricular systole (Figure 2.8).

Any condition in which right ventricular filling is limited, for example constrictive pericarditis, cardiac tamponade or right ventricular infarction, can cause elevation of the venous pressure which is more marked on inspiration when venous return to the heart increases. This rise in the JVP on inspiration, called Kussmaul's sign, is the opposite of what normally happens. This sign is best elicited with the patient sitting up at 90° and breathing quietly through the mouth.

Cannon a waves occur when the right atrium contracts against the closed tricuspid valve. This is usually a result of cardiac electrical abnormalities which have resulted in dissociation of atrial and ventricular contraction (e.g., complete heart block).

Large **v waves** occur in tricuspid regurgitation.

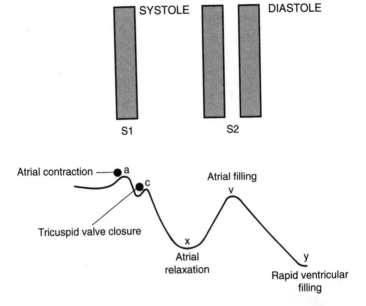

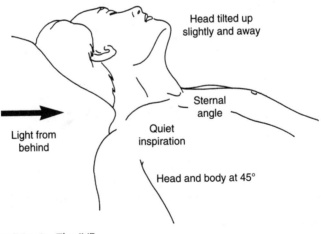

FIGURE 2.8 The JVP.

THE BACK

Percussion and auscultation of the lung bases (Chapter 3) are also part of the cardiovascular examination. Signs of cardiac failure may be detected in the lungs; in particular late or pan inspiratory crackles or a pleural effusion (usually left sided) may be present (Table 2.6). Remember that basal crackles are common and not always due to cardiac failure.

While the patient is sitting up, feel for pitting oedema of the sacrum (see below) which occurs in severe right heart failure, especially in patients who have been in bed.

THE ABDOMEN

Lie the patient down flat (on one pillow) and examine the abdomen (Chapter 4). The **liver** may become enlarged and tender due to

TABLE 2.6   Signs of Cardiac Failure (in approximate order of helpfulness)

Right Heart
Right ventricular third heart sound
Elevated jugular venous pressure (JVP)
Signs of tricuspid regurgitation — Large v waves, pulsatile liver
Peripheral oedema
Ascites

Left Heart
Third heart sound
Displaced and dyskinetic apex beat
Bilateral basal inspiratory crackles
Dyspnoea and especially orthopnoea (a symptom and a sign)
Pleural effusion (left or bilateral)

hepatic venous congestion in patients with right ventricular failure. This may be accompanied by **ascites** in severe cases.

THE LOWER LIMBS

Examine both femoral arteries (found by feeling in the inguinal crease about two-thirds of the way from the anterior superior iliac spine to the pubic tubercle), and then the arteries of the legs (Figure 2.9): the popliteal (behind the knee), posterior tibial (under the medial malleolus) and dorsalis pedis (on the forefoot) on both sides.

Palpate the distal shaft of the tibia for oedema by compressing the area gently for at least 15 seconds with the thumb. If **pitting** oedema is present, a little pit will appear in the shape of the examiner's thumb and refill only gradually.

Leg ulcers (which are typically on the medial side of the lower third of the leg above the medial malleolus when due to venous disease) and varicose veins should be noted. If varicose veins are present, the site of **venous valvular incompetence** should be determined. Examine for long saphenous incompetence as follows:

1. **Cough impulse test:** after standing the patient up, palpate just below the fossa ovalis (where the vein passes to join the femoral vein), which is 4 cm below and 4 cm lateral to the pubic tubercle, and ask the patient to cough. Feel for an impulse (thrill). Look also for a **saphena varix** (dilatation of the vein that produces a swelling in the fossa ovalis, which, unlike a femoral hernia disappears when the patient lies down).

2. **Trendelenberg's test:** after lying the patient down, elevate the (patient's) leg to empty the veins. Then compress the upper end of the vein in the groin with your hand and stand the patient up; if little or no filling occurs until the groin pressure is released sapheno-femoral valve incompetence is present and the test is positive. If filling occurs before the pressure is released, incompetent veins are in the thigh or calf.

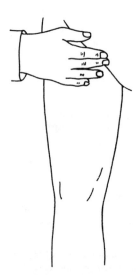

The femoral pulse is felt just below the inguinal ligament midway between the anterior superior iliac crest and the symphysis pubis

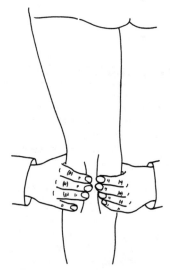

Popliteal artery – the leg is flexed to relax the hamstrings, and firm compression against the lower end of the tibial is applied

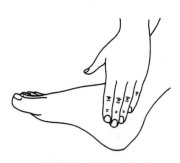

Posterior tibial artery is felt just behind the tip of the medial malleolus

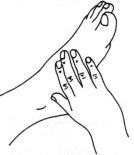

Dorsalis pedis is felt at the proximal end of the first intermetatarsal space

FIGURE 2.9   Sites of the peripheral pulses.

THE CARDIOVASCULAR SYSTEM — HINTS

1. Ischaemic heart disease should be suspected from the history. When angina is stable, the pain or discomfort occurs with a predictable amount of exertion and is relieved by rest. A recent increase in the frequency or the occurrence of pain at rest suggests unstable angina.

2. Cardiac dyspnoea (i.e., breathlessness due to cardiac failure) is worse on exertion or when the patient lies flat (orthopnoea).

3. Ask about cardiac risk factors for any patient with suspected cardiac disease; for example, smoking, known level of cholesterol and triglycerides, diabetes, family history of cardiac disease in first degree relatives.

4. Pay particular attention when examining the cardiovascular system to the rate, rhythm and character of the pulse, the level of the blood pressure, elevation of the jugular venous pressure, the position of the apex beat, and the presence of the heart sounds, any extra sounds or murmurs.

5. The position and timing of cardiac murmurs give important clues about the underlying valve lesion.

6. The most useful signs of left ventricular failure are a third heart sound a displaced and dyskinetic apex beat (Table 2.6).

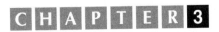

The chest

Chest: The trunk of the body, or cavity from the shoulders to the belly.

S JOHNSON, A DICTIONARY OF THE ENGLISH LANGUAGE (1755)

In this chapter, the symptoms and signs of lung disease are presented.

THE RESPIRATORY HISTORY

PRESENTING SYMPTOMS (Table 3.1)

Cough and Sputum

Cough is a common presenting respiratory symptom. Ask about the duration, whether it is dry or productive (i.e., of sputum), whether it is associated with wheeze and if the patient is taking any medications. Since the quality of the cough is important, ask the patient to describe the type of cough and to give a demonstration. A cough of recent origin, particularly if associated with fever and other symptoms of respiratory tract infection, may be due to acute bronchitis or pneumonia. A chronic cough associated with wheezing may be due to asthma; sometimes asthma can present with just cough alone. An irritating chronic dry cough can result from the reflux of acid into the oesophagus. A change in the character of a chronic cough may indicate the development of a new and serious underlying problem (e.g., infection or lung cancer).

A large volume of **purulent (yellow or green)** sputum suggests the diagnosis of **bronchiectasis** or **lobar pneumonia**. Foul-smelling dark coloured sputum may indicate the presence of a

67

TABLE 3.1 Respiratory History

Major Symptoms
   Cough
   Sputum
   Haemoptysis
   Dyspnoea (acute, progressive or paroxysmal)
   Wheeze
   Chest pain
   Fever
   Hoarseness
   Night sweats

lung abscess with anaerobic organisms. Pink frothy secretions from the trachea, which occur in pulmonary oedema, should not be confused with sputum. **Haemoptysis** (coughing up of blood) can be a sinister sign of lung disease and must always be investigated as it may be due to carcinoma of the lung, pneumonia, tuberculosis, pulmonary infarction or bronchiectasis.

Breathlessness (Dyspnoea)

Careful questioning about the timing of onset, severity and pattern of dyspnoea is helpful in making the diagnosis. Dyspnoea that is worse when the patient lies flat is more likely to be due to cardiac failure than a respiratory cause.

Dyspnoea can be graded from I to IV:

- Class I — dyspnoea on heavy exertion

- Class II — dyspnoea on moderate exertion

- Class III — dyspnoea on minimal exertion

- Class IV — dyspnoea at rest

It may be more useful, however, to determine the amount of exertion that is actually needed to cause dyspnoea, (i.e., the distance walked, or the number of steps climbed), or the ability to perform daily tasks such as dressing and washing.

Wheeze

A number of conditions can cause a continuous whistling noise during breathing (wheeze). These include asthma or chronic airflow limitation (chronic obstructive airways disease), and airway obstruction by a foreign body or tumour.

Chest Pain

Chest pain due to respiratory disease is characteristically pleuritic in nature (i.e., sharp and made worse by deep inspiration and coughing).

OTHER PRESENTING SYMPTOMS

Patients may occasionally present with episodes of **fever at night** (consider tuberculosis and pneumonia) or **hoarseness** (consider laryngitis, vocal cord tumour or recurrent laryngeal nerve palsy).

Patients with **obstructive sleep apnoea** (where airflow stops despite persistent respiratory efforts during sleep) typically present with daytime sleepiness (somnolence), chronic fatigue, morning headaches and personality disturbances. Very loud snoring may be reported by anyone within earshot.

Some patients respond to anxiety by increasing the rate and depth of their breathing. This is called **hyperventilation**. The resultant alkalosis may result in paraesthesia of the fingers and around the mouth, lightheadedness, chest pain and a feeling of impending collapse. Anxiety (e.g., during a panic attack) can also make patients feel that they need to take deep breaths.

PAST HISTORY

One should always ask about any previous respiratory illness including pneumonia, tuberculosis or chronic bronchitis, or abnormalities of the chest X-ray which have been previously reported to the patient.

TREATMENT

It is important to find out what drugs the patient is using, how often they are taken and whether they are inhaled or swallowed.

Almost every class of drug can produce lung toxicity. Examples include pulmonary embolism from use of the oral contraceptive pill, interstitial lung disease from cytotoxic agents, bronchospasm from beta-blockers or aspirin, and cough from ACE (angiotensin converting enzyme) inhibitors.

OCCUPATIONAL HISTORY

One must ask in some detail about possible exposure to dusts in mines and factories (e.g., asbestos, coal, silica, iron oxide, tin oxide, cotton, beryllium, titanium oxide, silver, nitrogen dioxide or anhydrides). Work or household exposure to animals, including birds, is also relevant (e.g., Q fever or psittacosis). Exposure to mouldy hay, humidifiers or air conditioners may also result in lung disease (e.g., allergic alveolitis). Exposure to spray painting and wood dusts may provoke occupational asthma, which may typically resolve on weekends or while on holidays.

SOCIAL HISTORY

A smoking history must be routine, as it is the major cause of chronic airflow limitation and lung cancer (Table 2.1). It is necessary to ask how many packets of cigarettes a day a patient has smoked and for how many years the patient has smoked.

FAMILY HISTORY

A family history of asthma, cystic fibrosis or emphysema should be sought. Alpha-1-antitrypsin deficiency, for example, is an inherited disease, in which case there may be a family history of emphysema.

EXAMINING THE CHEST

This should include a search for signs of lung disease, chest wall abnormalities and examination of the female breasts (see Chapter 8).

POSITIONING THE PATIENT

The patient should be undressed to the waist and, if well enough, should sit over the edge of the bed.

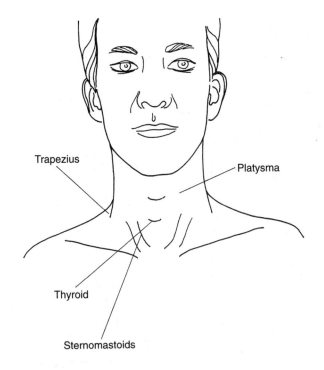

FIGURE 3.1   The accessory muscles of respiration.

GENERAL APPEARANCE

It is important to look for tachypnoea (a respiratory rate of more than 14 breaths a minute), use of the accessory muscles of respiration (sternomastoids, strap muscles and platysma, Figure 3.1) cyanosis and a spontaneous cough.

THE CHEST

The chest should be examined anteriorly and posteriorly by **inspection**, **palpation**, **percussion** and **auscultation**. Compare the right and left sides during each part of the examination.

Inspection

SHAPE AND SYMMETRY OF THE CHEST

When the anteroposterior (AP) diameter is increased compared with the lateral diameter, the chest is described as **barrel-shaped** (Figure 3.2a). An increase in the AP diameter indicates hyperinflation.

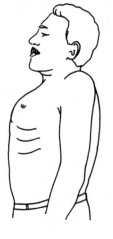

(a) Barrel shaped

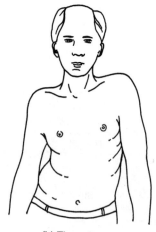

(b) Thoracic kyphoscoliosis

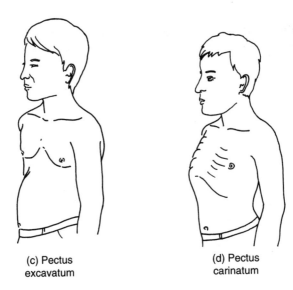

(c) Pectus
excavatum

(d) Pectus
carinatum

FIGURE 3.2   Chest shapes: (a) Barrel shaped (overexpanded),
(b) kyphosis, scoliosis, (c) pectus excavatum and
(d) pectus carinatum.

Kyphosis refers to an exaggerated forward curvature of the
spine, while **scoliosis** is lateral bowing (Figure 3.2b). Severe
thoracic kyphoscoliosis may reduce the lung capacity and
increase the work of breathing. Other quite common varieties in
chest shape include pectus encavatum (pidgeon chest) and
pectus carinatum (Figures 3.2c and 3.2d).

LESIONS OF THE CHEST WALL

These may or may not be obvious. Look for **scars** from previous
thoracic operations, or from chest drains inserted for a previous
pneumothorax or pleural effusion.

Radiotherapy for carcinoma of the lung or lymphoma may
cause erythema and thickening of the skin over the irradiated
area. There is a sharp demarcation between abnormal and normal
skin.

Subcutaneous emphysema is a crackling sensation felt on palpating the skin of the chest or neck. It is caused by air tracking from the lungs and is usually due to a pneumothorax.

Prominent veins may be seen in patients with superior vena caval obstruction.

MOVEMENT OF THE CHEST WALL

Look for **asymmetry** of chest wall movement anteriorly and posteriorly. Assessment of expansion of the **upper lobes** is best achieved by inspection from behind the patient, looking down at the clavicles during moderate respiration. The affected side will show delayed or decreased movement. For assessment of **lower lobe** expansion, the chest should be inspected posteriorly.

Reduced chest wall movement on one side may be due to localised pulmonary fibrosis, consolidation, collapse, pleural effusion or pneumothorax. Bilateral reduction of chest wall movement indicates a diffuse abnormality such as chronic airflow limitation or diffuse pulmonary fibrosis.

Palpation

CHEST EXPANSION

Place the hands firmly on the back of the chest wall with the fingers extending around the sides of the chest. The thumbs should almost meet in the middle line and should be lifted slightly off the chest so that they are free to move with respiration (Figure 3.3). As the patient takes a big breath in, the thumbs should move apart symmetrically at least 5 cm. Reduced expansion on one side indicates a lesion of the lobe on that side.

VOCAL FREMITUS

Palpate the chest wall with the palm of the hand while the patient repeats 'ninety-nine'. The front and back of the chest are each palpated in two comparable positions with the palm of one hand on each side of the chest. In this way differences in vibration on the chest wall can be detected. This can be a difficult sign to interpret. The causes of change in vocal fremitus are the same as those for vocal resonance (see page 81).

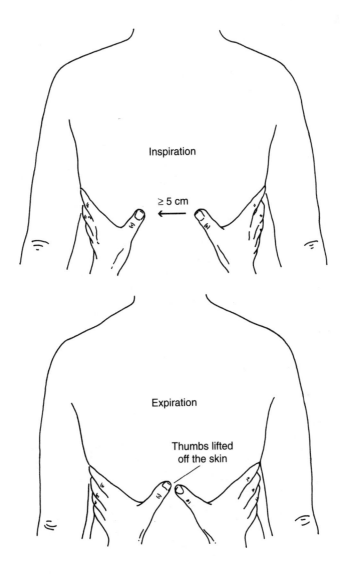

Inspiration

≥ 5 cm ←

Expiration

Thumbs lifted off the skin

FIGURE 3.3   Testing chest expansion.

RIBS

Gently compress the chest wall anteroposteriorly and laterally. Localised pain suggests a rib fracture, which may be secondary to trauma, or may be spontaneous as a result of tumour deposition or primary bone disease.

Percussion

With the left hand on the chest wall and the fingers slightly separated and aligned with the ribs, the middle finger is pressed firmly against the chest. Then the pad of the right middle finger is used to strike firmly the middle phalanx of the middle finger of the left hand. The percussing finger is quickly removed so that the note generated is not dampened. The percussing finger must be held partly flexed and a loose swinging movement should come from the wrist and not from the forearm (Figure 3.4). Percuss on both sides of the anterior, posterior and axillary regions and in the supraclavicular fossa over the apex of the lung. Percuss the clavicle directly with the percussing finger. For percussion posteriorly, the scapulae should be moved out of the way by asking the patient to move the elbows forward across the front of the chest (Figure 3.5).

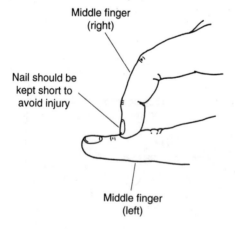

Middle finger
(right)

Nail should be
kept short to
avoid injury

Middle finger
(left)

FIGURE 3.4 Percussion technique.

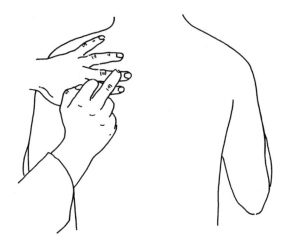

FIGURE 3.5 Percussing the back.

The feel of the percussion note is as important as its sound. The note is affected by the thickness of the chest wall, as well as by underlying structures. Percussion over a solid structure, such as the liver or a consolidated area of lung, produces a **dull** note. Percussion over a fluid-filled area, such as a pleural effusion, produces an extremely dull (**stony dull**) note. Percussion over the normal lung produces a resonant note and percussion over hollow structures, such as the bowel or a pneumothorax, produces a **hyper-resonant** note.

LIVER DULLNESS

The upper level of liver dullness is determined by percussing down the anterior chest in the mid-clavicular line. Normally, the upper level of the liver dullness is the fifth rib in the right mid-clavicular line. If the chest is resonant below this level it is a sign of hyperinflation, usually due to emphysema or asthma.

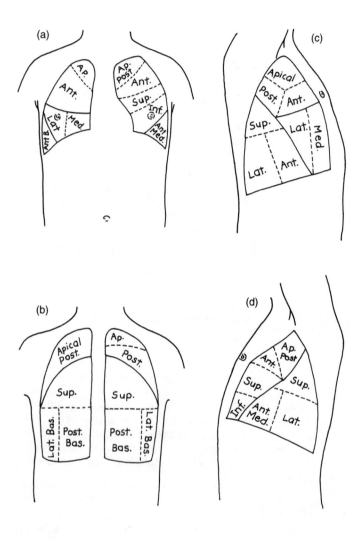

FIGURE 3.6 Surface markings of the lobes of the lungs and where to auscultate.

Auscultation

BREATH SOUNDS

Using the diaphragm of the stethoscope one should listen to the breath sounds in the areas shown in Figure 3.6. It is important to compare each side with the other. Remember to listen high up into the axillae and, using the bell of the stethoscope applied above the clavicles, to listen to the lung apices. Listen for the quality and intensity of the breath sounds and for the presence of additional (adventitious) sounds.

Quality of breath sounds: normal breath sounds are heard with the stethoscope over all parts of the chest. They had once been thought to arise in the alveoli (vesicles) of the lungs and are therefore called vesicular sounds. **Normal (vesicular)** breath sounds are **louder** and **longer** on **inspiration** than on expiration and there is no gap between the inspiratory and expiratory sounds (Figure 3.7).

Bronchial breath sounds: here turbulence in the large airways is heard without being filtered by the alveoli, producing a different sound. Bronchial breath sounds have a hollow, blowing quality. They are audible throughout expiration and there is often a gap between inspiration and expiration. The expiratory sound has a higher intensity and pitch than the inspiratory sound. They are heard over areas of consolidation since solid lung conducts the sound of turbulence in main airways to peripheral areas without filtering.

Intensity of the breath sounds: it is better to describe breath sounds as being of normal or reduced intensity than to speak about air entry.

Causes of reduced breath sounds include chronic airflow limitation, pleural effusion, pneumothorax, pneumonia, a large neoplasm, and pulmonary collapse.

Added (adventitious) sounds: there are two types of added sounds: continuous (wheezes) and interrupted (crackles).

Wheezes are usually the result of acute or chronic airflow obstruction due to asthma (often high pitched) or chronic airflow limitation (often low pitched).

Interrupted non-musical sounds are best called **crackles**.

Early inspiratory crackles of medium coarseness are characteristic of chronic airflow limitation. They are different from those heard in left ventricular failure, which occur later in the respiratory cycle.

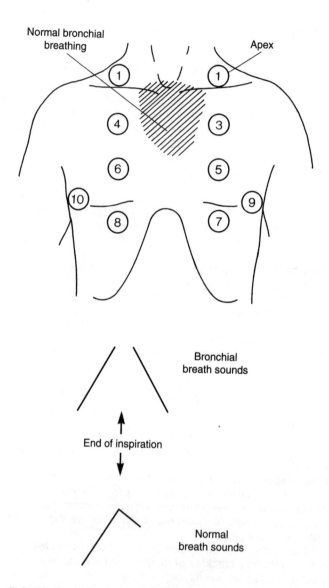

FIGURE 3.7 Character of normal and of bronchial breath sounds.

Late or pan-inspiratory crackles suggest disease confined to the alveoli. They may be fine, medium or coarse in quality.

Fine crackles have been likened to the sound of hair rubbed between the fingers or to the sound Velcro makes when being unstrapped — they are typically caused by pulmonary fibrosis.

Medium crackles are often due to left ventricular failure. They can also be present in patients with chronic airflow limitation.

Coarse crackles are characteristic of pools of retained secretions and have an unpleasant gurgling quality.

Pleural friction rub: when thickened, roughened pleural surfaces rub together as the lungs expand and contract; a continuous or intermittent grating sound may be audible. A pleural rub indicates pleurisy, which may be secondary to pulmonary infarction or pneumonia.

VOCAL RESONANCE

Auscultation over the chest while a patient speaks gives further information about the lungs' ability to transmit sounds. Over normal lung the low pitched components of speech are heard with a booming quality and high pitched components are attenuated.

Ask the patient to say 'ninety-nine' while you listen over each part of the chest. Over consolidated lung the numbers will become clearly audible while over normal lung the sound is muffled. If vocal resonance is present, bronchial breathing is likely to be heard.

THE HEART

Lie the patient at 45° and examine the jugular venous pressure for evidence of right heart failure. Next examine the praecordium with close attention to the pulmonary component of the second heart sound (P2). This is best heard at the second intercostal space on the left. It should not be louder than the aortic component, best heard at the right second intercostal space. If the P2 is louder, pulmonary hypertension should be strongly suspected.

PERIPHERAL SIGNS OF LUNG DISEASE

THE HANDS

Clubbing

Look for clubbing (page 28 and Figure 1.3) and its uncommon association, hypertrophic pulmonary osteoarthropathy (HPOA). Patients with HPOA have swelling and tenderness over the wrists and other involved areas. Respiratory causes of clubbing include carcinoma of the lung and chronic lung infection (e.g., pulmonary abscess, tuberculosis).

Staining

Look for staining of the fingers (actually caused by tar, as nicotine is colourless), a sign of cigarette smoking but not an indication of the number of cigarettes smoked.

Wasting and Weakness

Compression and infiltration by a peripheral lung tumour of a lower trunk of the brachial plexus results in wasting of the small muscles of the hand and weakness of finger abduction.

Pulse Rate

Tachycardia and pulsus paradoxus are important signs of severe asthma.

DYSPNOEA

Watch the patient for signs of dyspnoea at rest. Count the respiratory rate. Tachypnoea (>14 breaths a minute) means a rapid respiratory rate. Look to see whether the accessory muscles of respiration (the sternomastoids, the platysma and the strap muscles of the neck) are being used (Figure 3.1).

CYANOSIS

Look for central cyanosis by inspecting the tongue.

CHARACTER OF THE COUGH

Ask the patient to cough several times. Lack of the usual explosive beginning may indicate vocal cord paralysis (the 'bovine' cough). A muffled, wheezy ineffective cough suggests airflow limitation. A very loose productive cough suggests excessive bronchial secretions due to chronic bronchitis, pneumonia or bronchiectasis. A dry irritating cough may occur with chest infection, asthma or carcinoma of the bronchus and sometimes with left ventricular failure or interstitial lung disease.

Sputum

Note the volume and type (purulent, mucoid or mucopurulent). The presence or absence of blood should be recorded.

Stridor

Obstruction of the larynx, trachea or large airways may cause stridor, a rasping or croaking noise loudest on inspiration. This can be due to a foreign body, a tumour, infection (e.g., epiglottitis) or inflammation.

Hoarseness

Listen to the voice for hoarseness.

THE FACE

Inspect the **eyes** for evidence of Horner's syndrome where there is a constricted pupil and a partial ptosis (or closure of one eyelid) (page 139). This can be due to an apical lung tumour compressing the sympathetic nerves in the neck.

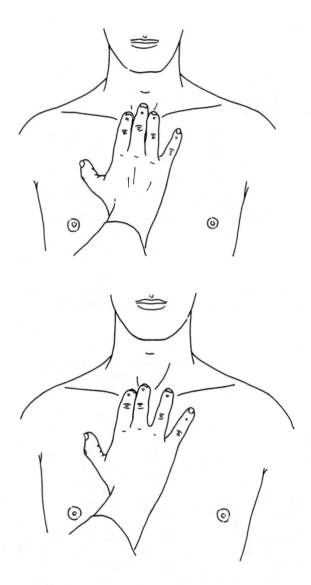

FIGURE 3.8 Feeling for the position of the trachea.

THE TRACHEA

From in front of the patient the forefinger of the right hand is pushed very gently up and backwards from the suprasternal notch until the trachea is felt. If the trachea is displaced to one side its edge rather than its middle will be felt and a larger space will be present on one side than the other (Figure 3.8). Slight displacement to the right is fairly common in normal people. This examination is uncomfortable for the patient so one must be gentle.

Significant displacement of the trachea suggests, but is not specific for, disease of the upper lobes of the lung.

Feel for a tracheal tug; the finger resting on the trachea feels it move inferiorly with each inspiration. This is a sign of gross overexpansion of the chest because of airflow obstruction.

THE CHEST HISTORY AND EXAMINATION — HINTS

1. Dyspnoea of respiratory cause can be difficult to distinguish from cardiac dyspnoea but orthopnea is not a feature of respiratory disease.

2. The smoking history and occupational history are particularly important in any patient with respiratory symptoms.

3. Production of sputum and particularly the presence of haemoptysis must be documented. Available sputum should be inspected.

4. Inspect for chest wall symmetry, palpate for expansion, percuss for dullness and auscultate for abnormal or reduced breath sounds. Examination of the upper lobes should not be forgotten.

5. It is useful to examine the posterior chest (lower lobes) first as in most cases 'this is where the money is' in respiratory disease.

6. Absence of clinical signs does not exclude a respiratory disease; the clinical signs can be less sensitive than investigations such as a chest X-ray (e.g., for detection of a mass lesion) or spirometry (e.g., airflow limitation).

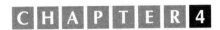

CHAPTER 4

The abdomen

*Gut: The long pipe stretching
with many convolutions from the
stomach to the vent.*

S JOHNSON, A DICTIONARY OF THE ENGLISH LANGUAGE (1775)

In this chapter an introduction to history taking and examination of conditions whose signs are found chiefly in the abdomen is presented. Gastrointestinal, haematological and renal disease can present with abdominal symptoms and signs and these are all discussed in this chapter.

THE GASTROINTESTINAL HISTORY

PRESENTING SYMPTOMS (Table 4.1)

Abdominal Pain

Careful history taking will often lead to the correct diagnosis of the cause of abdominal pain. The following aspects should be considered; **frequency** and **duration**, **severity**, **site** and **radiation**, **character** and **pattern**, **aggravating** and **relieving factors**, and **associated symptoms**.

FREQUENCY AND DURATION

Find out when the pain began and how often attacks have occurred. Abdominal pain may be acute or chronic.

TABLE 4.1 The Abdomen: Presenting Symptoms

GASTROINTESTINAL HISTORY

Major Symptoms

Abdominal pain
Appetite and/or weight change
Nausea and/or vomiting
Heartburn and/or acid regurgitation
Waterbrash
Dysphagia
Disturbed defaecation (diarrhoea, constipation, faecal
  incontinence)
Bleeding (haematemesis, melaena, rectal bleeding)
Jaundice
Dark urine, pale stools
Abdominal swelling
Pruritus
Lethargy
Fever

GENITOURINARY HISTORY

Major Symptoms

Change in appearance of urine, e.g., haematuria (red
  discolouration)
Change in urine volume or stream
— Polyuria (an increase in the volume of urine)
— Nocturia (getting up to pass urine during the
    night)
— Anuria (little or no urine output)
   Symptoms of prostatic enlargement
      Decrease in stream size
      Hesitancy
      Dribbling
      Urine retention
      Urinary frequency
      Urinary urgency (the need to pass urine
        without delay)
Incontinence of urine
Double voiding (incomplete bladder emptying)

TABLE 4.1 Continued

Renal colic
Symptoms of urinary infection:
    Dysuria (painful micturition), frequency (the need
        to pass small amounts of urine frequently),
        urgency, fever, loin pain
Urethral discharge
Symptoms suggestive of chronic renal failure
        (uraemia);
    Oliguria, nocturia, polyuria
    Anorexia, a metallic taste, vomiting, fatigue,
        hiccup, insomnia
    Itch, bruising, oedema
Impotence
Loss of libido
Infertility
Urethral or vaginal discharge
Genital rash
Menses
    Date of onset
    Regularity
    Last period (date)
    Dysmenorrhoea, menorrhagia, amenorrhoea
Pregnancies: number and any complications

HAEMATOLOGICAL HISTORY

Major Symptoms

Symptoms of anaemia: weakness, tiredness,
    dyspnoea, fatigue, postural dizziness
Bleeding (menstrual, gastrointestinal)
Easy bruising
Thrombotic tendency (e.g., repeated deep venous
    thrombosis in the legs)
Infection, fever or jaundice
Lymph gland enlargement
Bone pain
Paraesthesiae (e.g., B_{12} deficiency)
Skin rash
Weight loss
Night sweats

SEVERITY

Find out how much the pain interferes with normal activities.

SITE AND RADIATION

Ask the patient to point to the area affected and the site of maximum intensity. Ask if the pain travels elsewhere. Pain due to pancreatic disease or a penetrating peptic ulcer often radiates through to the back. Pain may radiate to the shoulder with diaphragmatic irritation or to the neck with oesophageal reflux.

CHARACTER AND PATTERN

Colicky pain comes and goes in waves and is related to peristaltic movements; it suggests bowel or ureteric obstruction. If the pain is chronic, one should ask if there is a daily pattern of pain.

AGGRAVATING AND RELIEVING FACTORS

Pain due to peptic ulceration may or may not be related to meals. Eating may precipitate ischaemic pain in the small bowel (mesenteric angina). Antacids or vomiting may relieve peptic ulcer pain or that of gastro-oesophageal reflux. Defaecation or passage of flatus may relieve the pain of colonic disease temporarily. Patients who get some relief by rolling around vigorously are more likely to have a colicky pain, while those who lie perfectly still are more likely to have peritonitis.

Patterns of Pain

PEPTIC ULCER DISEASE

This is classically a dull or burning pain in the epigastrium (see Figure 4.1) that is relieved by food or antacids and may occur postprandially. It is typically episodic and may occur at night, waking the patient from sleep. It is not possible to distinguish duodenal ulceration from gastric ulceration clinically.

PANCREATIC PAIN

This is often a steady, epigastric pain or ache which may be partly relieved by sitting up and leaning forward. There is often radiation of the pain to the back.

BILIARY PAIN

Although usually called 'biliary colic' this is rarely colicky; it is usually a severe constant right hypochondrial pain that can last for hours and occurs episodically. With cystic duct obstruction there is often epigastric pain. If cholecystitis develops, the pain typically shifts to the right upper quadrant and becomes more severe. The pain may also radiate across the upper abdomen and around to the right side of the back in the scapular region.

RENAL COLIC

This is a severe colicky pain superimposed on a background of constant pain in the renal angle, often with radiation towards the groin.

BOWEL OBSTRUCTION

Peri-umbilical pain suggests a small bowel origin but colonic pain can occur anywhere in the abdomen. Small bowel obstruction tends to cause more frequent colicky pain (with a cycle every 2 to 3 minutes) than large bowel obstruction (every 10 to 15 minutes). Obstruction is often associated with vomiting, constipation and abdominal distension.

Appetite or Weight Change

The presence of both anorexia (loss of appetite) and weight loss should make one suspicious of an underlying malignancy, but may also occur with depression or diabetes mellitus. The combination of weight loss with an increased appetite suggests malabsorption of nutrients or a hypermetabolic state (e.g., thyrotoxicosis).

Nausea and Vomiting

Nausea is the sensation of wanting to vomit. There are many gastrointestinal (e.g., peptic ulceration or gastric cancer causing pyloric outlet obstruction) and non-gastrointestinal (e.g., labyrinthitis, many drugs, migraine, renal failure) causes of nausea and vomiting. The volume and nature of the vomitus may suggest the cause of the problem. Vomiting of large volumes, but infrequently, suggests gastric outlet obstruction; the frequent vomiting of bile or faecal material, suggests bowel obstruction.

Heartburn and Acid Regurgitation

Heartburn refers to the presence of a burning pain or discomfort in the retrosternal area due to reflux of acid from the stomach into the oesophagus. Typically, this sensation travels up towards the throat and occurs after meals or is aggravated by bending, stooping or lying supine. Antacids usually relieve the pain at least transiently.

Acid regurgitation is an acid (sour) taste in the mouth which is due to reflux. **Waterbrash** refers to tasteless liquid (saliva) filling the mouth.

Dysphagia

Dysphagia is difficulty swallowing. Such difficulty may occur with solids or liquids. If a patient complains of difficulty swallowing, it is important to differentiate painful swallowing from actual difficulty. Painful swallowing is termed **odynophagia** and occurs with any severe inflammatory process involving the oesophagus.

If the patient complains of difficulty initiating swallowing or complains of fluid regurgitating into the nose or choking on trying to swallow, this suggests that the cause of the dysphagia is in the pharynx (**pharyngeal dysphagia**).

If the patient complains of food sticking after swallowing, it is important to consider causes of oesophageal blockage (e.g., carcinoma or stricture). If these patients also have symptoms of reflux, this suggests a stricture caused by oesophagitis. If there has been significant weight loss, this suggests cancer.

Diarrhoea

The symptom diarrhoea can be defined in a number of different ways. Patients may complain of frequent stools (more than three per day being abnormal) or they may complain of a change in the consistency of the stools which have become loose or watery.

When a history of diarrhoea is obtained, it is also important to determine if this has occurred acutely or whether it is a chronic problem. Acute diarrhoea is more likely to be infectious in nature while chronic diarrhoea has a large number of causes.

Consider, in chronic cases;

1. **Secretory diarrhoea:** the stools are of large volume (more than 1 litre a day) and the diarrhoea persists when the patient is fasting (e.g., due to a villous adenoma or a tumour secreting Vaso-active Intestinal Peptide (VIP).

2. **Osmotic diarrhoea:** the diarrhoea disappears when the patient fasts (e.g., due to taking a non-absorbed osmotic laxative).

3. **Exudative diarrhoea:** the stools are of small volume but frequent and there is associated blood or mucus (e.g., colon cancer or inflammatory bowel disease).

4. **Malabsorption:** if there is steatorrhoea (excess fat in the stools) the stools are pale, foul smelling and difficult to flush away.

5. **Increased intestinal motility** (e.g., thyrotoxicosis). Here the stools are normal in consistency and an increased bowel frequency may not be volunteered as a symptom.

Constipation

It is important to determine what patients mean if they say they are constipated. Constipation is a common symptom and can refer to the passage of infrequent stools (fewer than three times per week is abnormal), hard stools or stools that are difficult to evacuate. This symptom may occur acutely or may be a chronic problem.

Mucus

The passage of mucus (white flecks on the stool) may occur in inflammatory bowel disease, the irritable bowel syndrome, or with rectal carcinomas or villous adenomas.

Bleeding

Patients may present with haematemesis (vomiting blood), melaena (passage of jet black stools) or haematochezia (passage of bright red blood per rectum). Alternatively, with occult bleeding from the bowel they may present with symptoms and signs of anaemia (e.g., fatigue and pallor).

Jaundice

Usually the relatives notice a yellow discolouration of the sclera or skin due to bilirubin deposition before the patient does.

Ask about other symptoms including:

1. Abdominal pain; gallstones, for example, can cause biliary pain and jaundice.
2. Change in the colour of the stools and urine. Obstructive jaundice (e.g., blockage of the common bile duct by a gallstone) causes dark urine and pale stools while haemolytic anaemia is associated with dark urine and normal coloured stools.

PAST HISTORY

Ask about:

1. Surgical procedures, blood transfusions and anaesthetics.
2. Relapsing and remitting pain in the past (suggesting peptic ulceration) in a patient with sudden severe pain (perforated peptic ulcer).
3. A diagnosis of inflammatory bowel disease, and any treatment received.
4. Use of non-steroidal anti-inflammatory drugs (NSAIDs).

SOCIAL HISTORY

Ask about:

1. The patient's occupation.
2. Recent travel (e.g., to countries where hepatitis is endemic).
3. The alcohol intake.
4. Contact with people who have been jaundiced.
5. The use of intravenous drugs.

FAMILY HISTORY

A family history of bowel cancer, inflammatory bowel disease or liver disease is often relevant

THE GENITOURINARY HISTORY

PRESENTING SYMPTOMS (Table 4.1)

Patients may present with urinary tract symptoms (changes in the urine or in micturition), or abdominal or flank pain. Some patients have no symptoms but are found to be hypertensive or to have abnormalities on routine urinalysis or serum biochemistry.

Ask about: change in the appearance of the urine, symptoms of urinary obstruction (e.g., hesitancy, decrease in the size of the stream, terminal dribbling) and urinary incontinence. Ask about symptoms of renal failure: these are not specific but can include nocturia, anorexia, vomiting, fatigue, hiccup, insomnia and pruritus.

A menstrual history should always be obtained (including the date of menarche and the regularity of the menstrual cycle).

Ask about: Dysmenorrhoea (painful menstruation), menorrhagia (abnormally heavy periods), vaginal discharge, the number of pregnancies and births, complications of pregnancy and childbirth (e.g., hypertension) and contraceptive methods.

PAST HISTORY

Find out about recurrent urinary tract infections or calculi, renal surgery, any previous detection of proteinuria or microscopic haematuria, a diagnosis of diabetes mellitus, gout or hypertension, or the performance of a renal biopsy.

SOCIAL HISTORY

Ask about any social problems, and in renal failure patients about how the patient has coped and is coping with a serious chronic illness.

TREATMENT

A detailed drug history must be taken.

Find out if the patient is undergoing dialysis and whether this is haemodialysis or peritoneal dialysis.

A common form of treatment for renal failure is renal transplantation. A patient may be well informed about graft function, rejection episodes and drug treatment.

FAMILY HISTORY

Ask particularly about polycystic kidney disease, diabetes mellitus and hypertension in the family.

THE HAEMATOLOGICAL HISTORY

PRESENTING SYMPTOMS (Table 4.1)

Patients may present with symptoms of anaemia (e.g., lethargy, palpitations, dyspnoea on exertion or angina). Alternatively, the presenting symptoms may be of the condition leading to anaemia or of the causes of anaemia (e.g., rectal bleeding, or the bowel symptoms of malabsorption). The patient who complains of lymph node enlargement should be asked about sweats and weight loss (e.g., lymphoma). Recurrent infection may be the first symptom of a disorder of the immune system or of neutropenia. Patients with easy bruising or bleeding need a detailed history taken with questions about post-operative bleeding. If bleeding after trauma is immediate, this suggests a platelet problem; if bleeding occurs after a delay, a clotting factor problem is more likely.

PAST HISTORY

Ask about systemic disease and previous gastric surgery as causes of anaemia. Has the patient been refused as a blood donor, and if so, why?

TREATMENT

Find out about iron supplements or B_{12} injections, and use of NSAIDs, anticoagulants or chemotherapy. Find out if previous blood transfusions or venesections have been required.

FAMILY HISTORY

There may be a family history of thalassaemia, haemolytic anaemia (or jaundice), haemophilia or von Willebrand's disease.

EXAMINING THE ABDOMEN

INSPECTION

The patient should **lie flat** (Figure 4.1), with one pillow under the head and with the abdomen exposed from the nipples to the pubic symphysis. Inspection begins with a careful look for abdominal **scars** which may indicate previous surgery or trauma. Look in the area around the umbilicus for laparoscopic surgical scars. Older scars are white and recent scars are pink because the tissue remains vascular. Note the presence of **stomas** (colostomy, ileostomy or ileal conduit), fistulae or a peritoneal dialysis catheter. Nephrectomy scars are often more posterior than one might expect; they usually lie in the flank as far posterior as the erector spinae muscle group. Renal transplant scars are usually found in the right or left iliac fossae. A **transplanted kidney** may be visible as a bulge under the scar. Previous peritoneal dialysis results in small scars from catheter placement in the peritoneal cavity; these are situated on the lower abdomen, at or near the midline.

Generalised abdominal **distension** may be present. All the causes of this sound as if they begin with the letter 'F': fat (gross obesity), fluid (ascites), fetus, flatus (gaseous distension due to bowel obstruction), faeces, filthy big tumour (e.g., large polycystic kidneys or an ovarian tumour) or phantom pregnancy (looks pregnant but isn't). When the peritoneal cavity is filled with large volumes of fluid (ascites) from whatever cause, the abdominal flanks and wall appear tense and the umbilicus is shallow or everted and points downward.

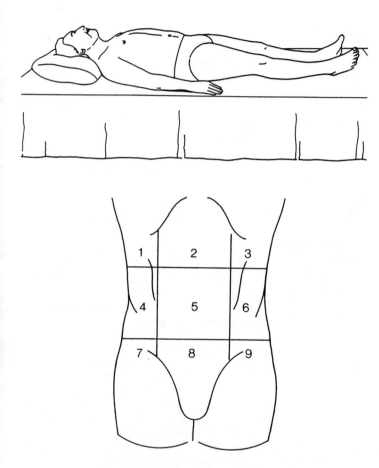

1. Right hypochondrium
2. Epigastrium
3. Left hypochondrium
4. Right lumbar region
5. Umbilical region
6. Left lumbar region
7. Right iliac fossa
8. Hypogastrium
9. Left iliac fossa

FIGURE 4.1 Abdominal examination: positioning the patient and the regions of the abdomen.

Local swellings may indicate enlargement of one of the abdominal or pelvic organs, or because of previous surgery weakening the abdominal wall (incisional hernia).

Prominent **veins** may be obvious on the abdominal wall in patients with severe portal hypertension or inferior vena cava obstruction.

Pulsations may be visible. An expanding central pulsation in the epigastrium suggests an abdominal aortic aneurysm. However, the abdominal aorta can often be seen to pulsate in normal thin people.

Visible peristalsis usually suggests intestinal obstruction.

Skin lesions should also be noted. These include the vesicles of herpes zoster, which occur in a radicular pattern (they are localised to only one side of the abdomen in the distribution of a single nerve root). Herpes zoster may be responsible for severe abdominal pain which is of mysterious origin until the rash appears.

Stretching of the abdominal wall severe enough to cause rupture of the elastic fibres in the skin produces pink linear marks with a wrinkled appearance which are called **striae**. When these are wide and purple-coloured, Cushing's syndrome (from steroid hormone excess) may be the cause. Ascites, pregnancy or recent loss of weight are much more common causes of striae.

Next, squat down beside the bed so that the patient's abdomen is at eye level. Ask him or her to take slow deep breaths through the mouth and watch for the movement of a large liver in the right upper quadrant (see below), or spleen in the left upper quadrant. Ask the patient to cough and look for the reducible swellings that indicate hernias. These may be present under scars (incisional hernias) or in the inguinal region.

PALPATION

Reassure the patient that the examination will not be painful and use warm hands. Ask if any particular area is tender and examine this area last.

For descriptive purposes the abdomen has been divided into nine areas or regions, or four quadrants (Figure 4.1). Palpation in each region is performed with the palmar surface of the fingers acting together. For the palpation of the edges of organs or masses the lateral surface of the forefinger is the most sensitive part of the hand.

Palpation should begin with **light pressure** in each region. Stop straight away if this causes pain. All the movements of the hand should occur at the metacarpophalangeal joints and the hand should be moulded to the shape of the abdominal wall. Note the presence of any tenderness or masses in each region.

Deep palpation of the abdomen is performed next. Deep palpation is used to detect deeper masses and to define those already discovered. Any mass must be characterised and described (Table 4.2).

Guarding of the abdomen, when resistance to palpation occurs due to contraction of the abdominal muscles, may result from tenderness or anxiety, and may be voluntary or involuntary. The latter suggests peritonitis. **Rigidity** is a constant involuntary contraction of the abdominal muscles always associated with tenderness and indicates peritoneal irritation. **Rebound tenderness** is said to be present when the abdominal wall, having been compressed slowly, is released rapidly and a sudden stab of pain results. This may make the patient wince so the face should be watched while this manoeuvre is performed. It strongly suggests the presence of peritonitis. If the abdomen is very tender, light percussion will give the same information and cause less discomfort.

The Liver

Feel for hepatomegaly (Figure 4.2). With the examining hand aligned parallel to the right costal margin, and beginning in the right iliac fossa, ask the patient to breathe in and out slowly through the mouth. With each expiration the hand is advanced by 1 or 2 cm closer to the right costal margin. During inspiration the hand is kept still and the lateral margin of the forefinger waits expectantly for the liver edge to strike it.

If the liver is palpable, its surface should be felt. The edge of the liver and the surface itself may be;

1. hard or soft

2. tender or non-tender

3. regular or irregular

4. pulsatile or non-pulsatile.

TABLE 4.2   Descriptive Features of Intra-abdominal Masses

For any abdominal mass all the following should be determined.

1. Site: the region involved and depth (e.g., abdominal wall, intra-abdominal or retroperitoneal)

2. Tenderness

3. Size (which must be measured) and shape

4. Surface, which may be regular or irregular

5. Edge, which may be regular or irregular

6. Consistency, which may be hard or soft

7. Mobility and movement with inspiration

8. Whether it is pulsatile or not

9. Whether one can get above the mass

The normal liver edge may be palpable just below the right costal margin on deep inspiration, especially in thin people. The edge is then felt to be soft and regular with a fairly sharply defined border and the surface of the liver itself is smooth.

If the liver edge is palpable the total **liver span** should be measured. The normal upper border of the liver is level with the fifth rib in the midclavicular line. At this point the percussion note

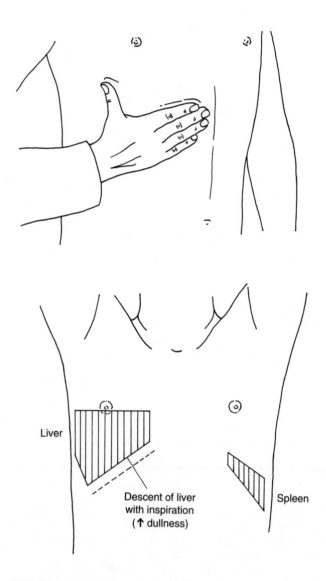

FIGURE 4.2 Abdominal examination: the liver.

over the chest changes from resonant to dull. To estimate the liver span, percuss down along the right midclavicular line until the liver dullness is encountered and measure from here to the palpable liver edge. The normal span is 12–15 cm.

The Gallbladder

The gallbladder is occasionally palpable below the right costal margin where this crosses the lateral border of the rectus muscles but this does not occur in health. If biliary obstruction or gall bladder disease is suspected, the examining hand should be oriented perpendicular to the costal margin, feeling from medial to lateral. Unlike the liver edge, the gallbladder if palpable will be a bulbous, focal rounded mass which moves downwards on inspiration.

Murphy's sign should be sought if cholecystitis is suspected. While taking a deep breath in, the patient catches his or her breath when an inflamed gallbladder presses on the examiner's hand which is lying at the costal margin.

The Spleen

The spleen enlarges inferiorly and medially. Its edge should be sought below the umbilicus in the midline initially. A two-handed technique is recommended (Figure 4.3). The left hand is placed posterolaterally just below the left lower ribs and the right hand is placed on the abdomen parallel to the left costal margin. Don't start palpation too near the costal margin or a large spleen will be missed. As the right hand is advanced closer to the left costal margin, the left hand compresses firmly over the rib cage so as to produce a loose fold of skin; this removes tension from the abdominal wall and enables a slightly enlarged soft spleen to be felt as it moves down towards the right iliac fossa at the end of inspiration.

If the spleen is not palpable, the patient must be rolled on to the right side towards the examiner and palpation repeated. Here one begins close to the left costal margin.

The Kidneys

An attempt to palpate the kidney should be a routine part of the examination. Use a **bimanual method**. The patient lies flat on his

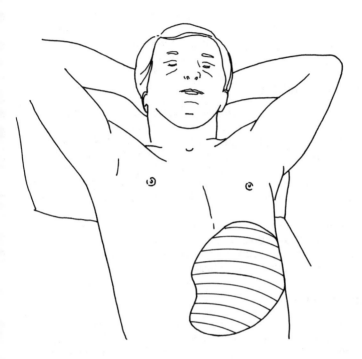

FIGURE 4.3 The spleen: bimanual palpation with the patient
rolled towards the examiner.

or her back. To palpate the right kidney, the examiner's left hand
slides underneath the back to rest with the heel of the hand under
the right loin. The fingers remain free to flex at the metacarpophalangeal joints in the area of the renal angle. The flexing
fingers can push the contents of the abdomen anteriorly. The
examiner's right hand is placed over the right upper quadrant
(Figure 4.4).

When the clinician ballotts the kidneys, the renal angle is
pressed sharply by the flexing fingers of the posterior hand. The
kidney can be felt to float upwards and strike the anterior hand.
The opposite hands are used to palpate the left kidney.

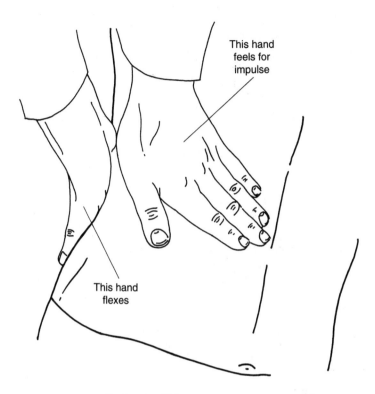

This hand
feels for
impulse

This hand
flexes

FIGURE 4.4   Ballotting the kidneys.

The lower pole of the right kidney (Figure 4.4) may be palpable in thin, normal persons. Both kidneys move downwards only a little with inspiration.

It is particularly common to confuse a large left kidney with an enlarged spleen. The major distinguishing features are:

1. The spleen has no palpable upper border — one cannot feel the space between the spleen and the costal margin, which is present in renal enlargement.

2. The spleen, unlike the kidney, has a notch anteromedially which may be palpable.

3. The spleen moves inferomedially on inspiration while the kidney moves inferiorly.

4. The spleen is not usually ballottable unless gross ascites is present, but the kidney is, again because of its retroperitoneal position.

5. The percussion note is dull over the spleen but is usually resonant over the kidney, as the latter lies posterior to loops of gas-filled bowel.

6. A friction rub may occasionally be heard over the spleen, but never over the kidney because it is too posterior.

PERCUSSION

Percussion is used to define the size and nature of organs and masses and to detect fluid in the peritoneal cavity. It is more reliable for the detection of an enlarged liver than for an enlarged spleen.

Ascites

Routine abdominal examination should include percussion starting in the midline with the finger pointing towards the feet; the percussion note is tested out towards the flanks on each side (Figure 4.5).

If dullness in the flanks is detected the sign of **shifting dullness** should be sought. The clinician stands on the right side of the bed and percusses out to the left flank until dullness is reached. This point should be marked with a finger or a pen (not an indelible one) and the patient rolled towards the examiner. After 30 seconds or so percussion is repeated over the marked point.

Shifting dullness is present if the area of dullness has changed to become resonant.

AUSCULTATION

Bowel Sounds

Place the diaphragm of the stethoscope just below the umbilicus. Bowel sounds can be heard over all parts of the abdomen in

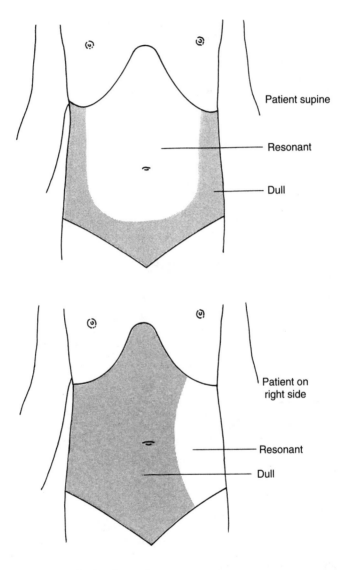

Patient supine

Resonant

Dull

Patient on
right side

Resonant

Dull

FIGURE 4.5 Testing for ascites.

normal healthy people. They have a soft gurgling character and occur only intermittently. Bowel sounds should be described as either **present** or **absent**.

Complete absence of bowel sounds over a three-minute period indicates **paralytic ileus**.

The bowel that is obstructed produces a louder and more high pitched sound with a **tinkling** quality which is due to the presence of air and liquid ('obstructed bowel sounds'). Intestinal hurry or rush, which may occur in diarrhoeal states, causes loud gurgling sounds (borborygmi) which are often audible without the stethoscope.

THE GROIN

Examine the inguinal nodes, look for hernias and palpate the testes.

INGUINAL LYMPH NODES

There are two groups — one along the inguinal ligament and the other along the femoral vessels. A method of characterising palpable lymph nodes is summarised in Table 4.3. Small (<1 cm diameter), firm mobile nodes are commonly found in normal people.

HERNIAS

In the patient with an acute abdomen, a strangulated hernia must be excluded as a cause in all cases. If a hernia is not obvious while the patient is lying down, complete examination requires that the patient be examined while standing.

Inguinal Hernias

First decide if the swelling in the groin is above or below the inguinal ligament, which lies between the anterior superior iliac spine and the pubic tubercle. The pubic tubercle is found just above the attachment of the adductor longus tendon to the pubic bone, which can be felt on the upper medial aspect of the thigh. If

TABLE 4.3 Characteristics of Lymph Nodes

During the palpation of lymph nodes the following features must be considered:

Site
Palpable nodes may be localised to one region (e.g., local infection, early lymphoma) or be generalised (e.g., late lymphoma)

The palpable lymph node areas are:
    epitrochlear
    axillary
    cervical (includes occipital and
    supraclavicular)
    para-aortic (rarely palpable)
    inguinal
    popliteal

Size
Large nodes are usually abnormal (greater than 1 cm)

Consistency
Hard nodes suggest carcinoma deposits, soft nodes may be normal, and rubbery nodes may be due to lymphoma

Tenderness
This implies infection or acute inflammation

Fixation
Nodes that are fixed to underlying structures are more likely to be infiltrated by carcinoma than mobile nodes

Overlying Skin
Inflammation of the overlying skin suggests infection, and tethering to the overlying skin suggests carcinoma

the swelling lies **medial** to and **above** the pubic tubercle it is likely to be an inguinal hernia (Figure 4.6). The characteristic inguinal hernia is a soft lump which can usually be pushed back into the abdominal cavity (i.e., is reducible) and an impulse is palpable if the patient coughs. The cough impulse must always be sought.

An **indirect inguinal hernia** passes through the internal inguinal ring, which lies 2 cm above the mid point of the inguinal ligament, just above and lateral to the femoral pulse and descends through the inguinal canal. In males a small indirect inguinal hernia may be palpated by gently invaginating the scrotum and feeling an impulse at the external ring when the patient coughs. Remember that, when examining a male, one should count the number of testes in the scrotum (normally two) as a maldescended testis may be confused with an inguinal hernia.

Direct inguinal hernias, protrude forward through the inguinal (Hesselbach's) triangle. A direct inguinal hernia usually appears immediately with standing (and coughing or straining) and disappears on lying down.

Femoral Hernias

These occur **lateral** to and **below** the pubic tubercle, 2 cm medial to the femoral pulse, and do not involve the inguinal canal. There may not be a cough impulse because of the presence of an omental plug or strangulation. Do not confuse an impulse conducted by the femoral vein (saphena varix) during coughing with a femoral hernia. A femoral hernia is usually small and firm and can be mistaken for a lymph node.

If a hernia strangulates the overlying skin may become red and tense, and the lump is usually tender. The cough impulse is lost. Remember that hernias are often bilateral, that two different types may occur on the same side, and that there may be an associated hydrocele (one can get above a hydrocele in the inguinal canal but not a hernia).

Incisional Hernias

Any abdominal scar may be the site of a hernia because of abdominal wall weakness. Assess this by asking the patient to cough while you look for abnormal bulges. Next have the patient

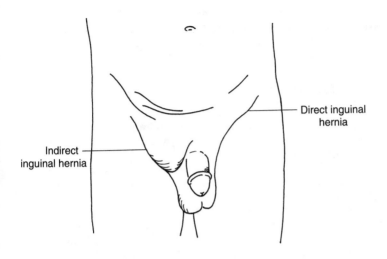

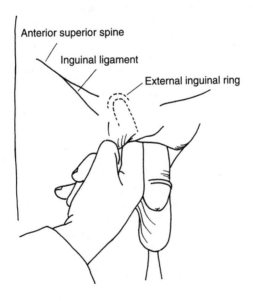

FIGURE 4.6   Inguinal hernias.

lift the head and shoulders off the bed while the examiner's hand rests on the forehead and resists this movement. If a bulge is seen the examiner's other hand should palpate for a fascial layer defect in the muscle.

MALE GENITALIA

Palpate the scrotum for the **testes**. The **spermatic cord** is palpable as it enters the scrotum: the **epididymis** on top of each testis is also usually palpable.

Inspect the scrotum for size and skin changes (e.g., ulceration). Feel each testis rather gently and note the size, regularity and firmness. There may be a mass in the scrotum separate from the testes. If it is not possible to find the upper limit of this mass it must have descended into the testis from above and is probably an inguinal hernia. A mass wholly within the testis should be tested for transillumination (Figure 4.7) with a torch. A hydrocele is confined to the scrotum, will usually light up in an impressive manner, and the testis and epididymis are not palpable.

Bilateral **testicular atrophy** occurs in chronic liver disease (e.g., alcoholic liver disease, haemochromatosis).

RECTAL EXAMINATION

The abdominal examination is not complete without the performance of a rectal examination. Following an explanation as to what is to happen, the patient lies on his or her left side with the knees drawn up and back to the examiner. This is called the left lateral position.

The examiner dons a pair of gloves and begins the inspection of the anus and perianal area by separating the buttocks. Note the presence of thrombosed external haemorrhoids (piles: small (less than 1 cm), tense bluish swellings seen on one side of the anal margin) or skin tags (these look like tags elsewhere on the body and can be an incidental finding or occur with haemorrhoids or Crohn's disease). Symptoms or signs of an acute anal fissure precludes a rectal examination as it would cause the patient severe pain.

The tip of the gloved right index finger is lubricated and placed over the anus. Ask the patient to breathe in and out quietly through

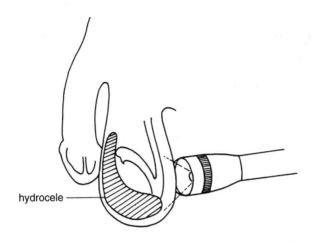

hydrocele

FIGURE 4.7 Transillumination of the testes.

the mouth, as a distraction and to aid relaxation. Slowly increasing pressure is applied with the pulp of the finger until the sphincter is felt to relax slightly. The finger is then advanced into the rectum slowly. At this stage external sphincter tone should be assessed as increased, normal or reduced.

Palpation of the anterior wall of the rectum for the **prostate gland** in the male and for the **cervix** in the female is performed first. The normal prostate is a firm rubbery bi-lobed mass with a central furrow. The presence of a very hard nodule suggests carcinoma of the prostate is present. The prostate is boggy and tender in patients with prostatitis. A mass above the prostate or cervix may indicate a metastatic deposit on Blumer's shelf. The finger is then rotated clockwise so that the left lateral wall, posterior wall and right lateral wall of the rectum can be palpated in turn. Then the finger is advanced as high as possible into the rectum and slowly withdrawn along the rectal wall. After the finger has been withdrawn the glove is inspected for bright blood or melaena, mucus or pus, and the colour of the faeces is noted. Haemorrhoids are not palpable unless thrombosed. The occurrence of significant pain during the examination suggests an anal fissure, an ischiorectal abscess, a recently thrombosed external haemorrhoid, proctitis or anal ulceration.

OTHER SIGNS IN ABDOMINAL DISEASE

GENERAL INSPECTION

Look for jaundice (yellow sclerae), increased pigmentation (e.g., haemochromatosis), obesity or wasting (record the weight and height). Wasting may be due to malabsorption or malignancy (Table 4.4).

Note any rashes. Fragile vesicles appear on exposed areas of the skin and heal with scarring in patients with porphyria cutanea tarda. The tense tethering of the skin in systemic sclerosis may be

TABLE 4.4 Assessing the Patient with Suspected Malignancy

1. Palpate all draining lymph nodes

2. Examine all remaining lymph node groups

3. Examine the abdomen, particularly for hepatomegaly and ascites

4. Feel the testes

5. Perform a rectal examination and pelvic examination

6. Examine the lungs

7. Examine the breasts

8. Examine the skin and nails for melanoma

associated with gastro-oesophageal reflux and gastrointestinal motility disorders.

Look for the general signs of uraemia including hyperventilation (metabolic acidosis), hiccupping, uraemic fetor (the breath smells rather like that of urine) and a sallow complexion.

Assess the state of hydration in all patients with suspected renal disease. Dehydration can be a cause of acute renal failure while overhydration can result from intravenous infusions of fluid when attempts are made to correct acute renal failure.

NAILS

Leuconychia (White Nails)

When chronic liver or other disease results in hypoalbuminaemia, the nail beds opacify, often leaving only a rim of pink nail bed at the top of nail.

Clubbing

Of patients with cirrhosis, up to one-third may have finger clubbing.

Koilonychia

These are dry, brittle, ridged, spoon-shaped nails due to severe iron deficiency anaemia.

THE HANDS

Note any changes of **arthritis**. Arthropathy may be present in the hands in patients with the iron storage disease, **haemochromatosis**.

Look for **purpura**, which is really any sort of bruising. The lesions can vary in size from pinheads called petechiae to large bruises called ecchymoses.

If the petechiae are raised (**palpable purpura**), this suggests an underlying systemic vasculitis or bacteraemia.

At the **wrist** and **forearms** inspect for **scars** and palpate for surgically created **arteriovenous fistulae** or **shunts**, used for haemodialysis access. There is a longitudinal swelling and a palpable continuous thrill present over the fistula.

THE PALMS

Palmar Erythema ('Liver Palms')

This is reddening of the palms of the hands affecting the thenar and hypothenar eminences. Often the soles of the feet are also affected. This can be a feature of chronic liver disease.

Anaemia

Inspect the palmar creases for pallor suggesting anaemia which may result from gastrointestinal blood loss, malabsorption (folate, vitamin B_{12}), haemolysis (e.g., hypersplenism) or chronic systemic disease.

Dupuytren's Contracture

This is a visible and palpable thickening and contraction of the palmar fascia causing permanent flexion, most often of the ring finger. It is often bilateral and occasionally may affect the feet. It is associated with alcoholism (not liver disease), but is also found in some manual workers; it may be familial.

HEPATIC FLAP (ASTERIXIS)

Ask the patient to stretch out the arms in front, separate the fingers and extend the wrists for 15 seconds. Jerky, irregular flexion-extension movement at the wrist and metacarpophalangeal joints, often accompanied by lateral movements of the fingers, constitute the flapping of hepatic encephalopathy in liver failure.

THE ARMS

Inspect the upper limbs for **bruising**. Large bruises (ecchymoses) may be due to clotting abnormalities (e.g., in chronic liver disease).

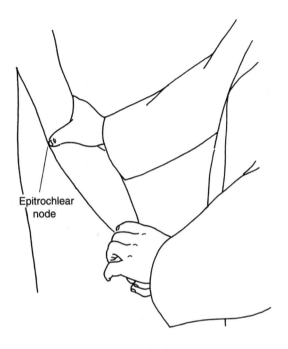

FIGURE 4.8   Feeling for the epitrochlear lymph node.

Look for muscle wasting which is often a late manifestation of malnutrition in alcoholic patients. Alcohol can also cause a proximal myopathy (page 162).

Scratch marks due to severe itch (pruritus) are often prominent in patients with obstructive or cholestatic jaundice.

Examine the **epitrochlear nodes**. Place the palm of the right hand under the patient's right elbow. The examiner's thumb can then be placed over the node which is proximal and slightly anterior to the medial epicondyle. This is repeated with the left hand for the other side (Figure 4.8).

Spider naevi consist of a central arteriole from which radiate numerous small vessels which look like spiders' legs. They range in size from just visible to half a centimetre in diameter. Their usual distribution is in the area drained by the superior vena cava, so

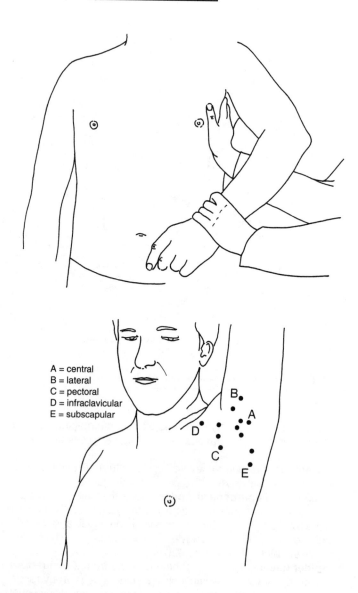

A = central
B = lateral
C = pectoral
D = infraclavicular
E = subscapular

FIGURE 4.9   Feeling for the axillary lymph nodes.

they are found on the arms, neck and chest wall. Pressure applied with a pointed object to the central arteriole causes blanching of the whole lesion. Rapid refilling occurs on release of the pressure.

The finding of more than two spider naevi anywhere on the body is likely to be abnormal except during pregnancy. Spider naevi can be caused by cirrhosis, most frequently due to alcohol.

They can easily be distinguished from **Campbell de Morgan spots** which are flat or slightly elevated red circular spots which occur on the abdomen or the front of the chest. They do not blanch on pressure and are very common and harmless.

AXILLAE

The axillary lymph nodes are palpated by raising the patient's arm and, using the left hand for the right side, the examiner pushes his or her fingers as high as possible into the axilla. The patient's arm is then brought down to rest on the examiner's forearm. The opposite is done for the other side (Figure 4.9).

There are five main groups of axillary nodes: (i) central; (ii) lateral (above and lateral); (iii) pectoral (medial); (iv) infra-clavicular; and (v) subscapular (most inferior). An effort should be made to feel for nodes in each of these areas of the axilla.

CERVICAL AND SUPRACLAVICULAR NODES
(Table 4.3)

Sit the patient up and examine the cervical nodes from behind. There are eight groups. Attempt to identify each of the groups of nodes with your fingers (Figure 4.10). Palpate first the submental node which lies directly under the chin, then the submandibular nodes which are below the angle of the jaw. Next palpate the jugular chain which lies anterior to the sternomastoid muscle and then the posterior triangle nodes which are posterior to the sternomastoid muscle. Palpate the occipital region for occipital nodes and then move to the postauricular node behind the ear and the preauricular node in front of the ear. Finally from the back, with the patient's shoulders slightly shrugged, feel in the supra-clavicular fossa and at the base of the sternomastoid muscle for the supraclavicular nodes.

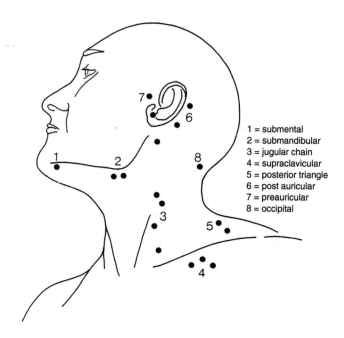

1 = submental
2 = submandibular
3 = jugular chain
4 = supraclavicular
5 = posterior triangle
6 = post auricular
7 = preauricular
8 = occipital

FIGURE 4.10 The cervical nodes.

THE FACE

Eyes

Look first at the sclerae for signs of **jaundice** or **anaemia**. **Iritis** (page 167) may be seen in inflammatory bowel disease.

Conjunctival pallor suggests anaemia and is more reliable than examination of the nailbeds or palmar creases.

The Salivary Glands (Figure 4.11)

The normal **parotid gland** is impalpable; enlargement leads to a swelling in the cheek behind the angle of the jaw and in the upper

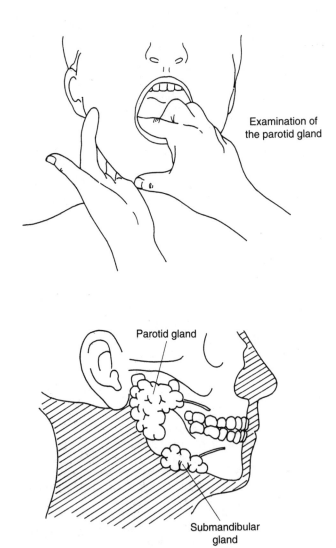

Examination of
the parotid gland

Parotid gland

Submandibular
gland

FIGURE 4.11 The salivary glands.

neck. Examine for signs of inflammation (warmth, tenderness, redness and swelling) and decide if the facial swelling is lumpy or not. Alcoholic liver disease can cause bilateral swelling. A mixed parotid tumour (a pleomorphic adenoma) is the commonest cause of a lump. Parotid carcinoma may cause a facial nerve palsy (page 143). Feel in the mouth for a parotid calculus which may be present at the parotid duct orifice (opposite the upper second molar). Mumps also causes acute parotid enlargement which is usually bilateral.

Submandibular gland enlargement is most often due to a calculus. This may be palpable bimanually. The examiner's index finger is placed on the floor of the mouth beside the tongue, feeling between it and fingers placed behind the body of the mandible (wear a glove!). It may also be enlarged in chronic liver disease.

The Mouth

THE TEETH AND BREATH

Look first briefly at the state of the teeth and note whether they are real or false. False teeth will have to be removed for complete examination of the mouth. Loose-fitting false teeth may be responsible for ulcers and decayed teeth may be responsible for fetor.

Fetor hepaticus is a sweet smell of the breath. It is an indication of hepatocellular failure.

THE TONGUE

Thickened epithelium with bacterial debris and food particles commonly cause a **coating** over the tongue, especially in smokers. It is rarely a sign of disease.

Leucoplakia is white coloured thickening of the mucosa of the tongue and mouth; the condition is premalignant. Most of the causes of leucoplakia begin with 'S': sore teeth (poor dental hygiene), smoking, spirits, sepsis or syphilis, but often no cause is apparent.

The term '**glossitis**' is generally used to describe a smooth appearance of the tongue which may also be erythematous. The appearance is due to atrophy of the papillae, and in later stages there may be shallow ulceration. These changes occur in the tongue often as a result of nutritional deficiencies (e.g., Vitamin B_{12}, folate or iron).

ORAL CAVITY

Aphthous ulceration is common. It begins as a small painful vesicle on the tongue or mucosal surface of the mouth which may break down to form a painful shallow ulcer with surrounding erythema. These ulcers heal without scarring. They usually do not indicate any serious underlying systemic disease, but may occur in Crohn's disease or coeliac disease.

Fungal infection with **Candida albicans** (thrush) causes creamy white curd-like patches in the mouth or tongue which are removed only with difficulty and leave a bleeding surface.

Look for hypertrophy of the gums, which may occur with infiltration by leukaemic cells especially in acute monocytic leukaemia and for gum bleeding, ulceration, infection and haemorrhage of the buccal and pharyngeal mucosa. Also look for telangiectasia (which may be a sign of hereditary haemorrhagic telangiectasia that causes occult bleeding in the bowel).

THE CHEST

In males, **gynaecomastia** or enlargement of the breasts may be a sign of chronic liver disease.

THE BACK

Strike the vertebral column gently with the base of the fist to elicit bony tenderness. This may be due to malignant deposits. Look for sacral oedema in a patient confined to bed, (e.g., from nephrotic syndrome or congestive cardiac failure).

THE LEGS

Note oedema, purpura, pigmentation or scratch marks (**pruritus** [itch] may be associated with renal failure and obstructive jaundice because toxins are deposited in the skin).

Leg ulcers may occur above the medial or lateral malleolus in association with haemolytic anaemia (including sickle cell anaemia and hereditary spherocytosis).

Look for the neurological signs of alcoholism (e.g., a coarse tremor) or evidence of thiamine deficiency (peripheral neuropathy or memory loss) may also be present (page 130).

THE FUNDI

Look for engorged retinal vessels and papilloedema (page 170). This can occur in diseases such as macroglobulinaemia which increase blood viscosity. Haemorrhages may occur with severe thrombocytopenia, especially when it is associated with anaemia.

URINALYSIS

The urine should be tested with a dip stick for certain abnormalities and for pH. Colour changes on the stick will indicate pH, protein (proteinuria), sugar diabetes mellitus, nitrites (possible infection) and red blood cells (haematuria).

THE ABDOMINAL HISTORY AND EXAMINATION — HINTS

1. Eliciting the individual gastrointestinal symptoms and the pattern of presentation will often lead to the correct diagnosis.

2. The symptoms and signs of renal disease may be non-specific and a thorough history and examination is required.

3. Abnormal bruising or bleeding tendencies may have been noticed and should be asked about.

4. When examining the abdomen, it is important to position the patient flat. While palpating, consider the underlying organs that are present when abnormalities are detected.

5. A left upper quadrant mass may be a spleen or kidney. Remember that one cannot get above the spleen and that the spleen is not ballottable.

6. Lymphadenopathy is a major sign of haematological disease and all lymph node groups must be carefully examined.

7. A gastrointestinal system examination is incomplete without a rectal examination.

8. Examination of the urine is an extension of the physical examination and should not be omitted.

9. Assessing a patient with a suspected malignancy includes a careful routine of examination (Table 4.4).

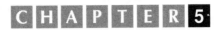

The nervous system

Brain: that collection of vessels and organs in the head, from which sense and motion arise

S JOHNSON, A DICTIONARY OF THE ENGLISH LANGUAGE (1775)

Neurological history and examination require an approach that is very systematic and thorough. Only by this means can the symptoms and signs be assembled in a way that will enable a sensible neurological diagnosis.

THE NEUROLOGICAL HISTORY

(Table 5.1)

The **temporal course of a neurological illness** may give important information about the underlying aetiology. An acute onset of symptoms suggests a vascular problem, a subacute onset suggests an inflammatory disorder, while a more chronic symptom course suggests that the underlying disorder may be related to either a tumour or a degenerative process. Metabolic or toxic disorders may present with any of these patterns.

A judgment must also be made as to whether the disease process is **localised or diffuse**, and what **levels of the nervous system** are involved.

HEADACHE AND FACIAL PAIN

Headache is a common and difficult symptom but the diagnosis may be clear once the pattern has been determined.

127

Tension-type headache may be episodic or chronic, commonly bilateral, and occurs over the frontal, occipital or temporal areas. It may be described as a sensation of tightness. These headaches last for hours, recur often and lack the specific features of other headaches. It is the commonest type.

Classical migraine is usually a unilateral headache that is preceded by an aura (e.g., flashing lights) and is commonly associated with photophobia (light intolerance). It is often of incapacitating severity and associated with nausea and vomiting. **Common migraine** is a similar headache without the other neurological symptoms and is much more common.

Cluster headache is a severe steady boring pain behind or over one eye lasting 15 minutes to 2 hours, associated with lacrimation, rhinorrhoea and flushing of the forehead. It tends to occur at the same time each day, often at night.

Cervical spondylosis causes headache over the occiput which is associated with neck pain.

Raised intracranial pressure results in generalised headache that is worse in the morning and may be associated with drowsiness or vomiting and progressive neurological deficits.

Meningitis causes generalised headache associated with photophobia, fever and a stiff neck.

Temporal arteritis causes persistent headache usually over the temporal area associated with tenderness over the temporal artery. There may be jaw claudication (pain on eating or talking) as well as acute visual loss.

Acute sinusitis headache is associated with pain or fullness behind the eyes or over the cheeks or forehead.

Subarachnoid haemorrhage characteristically causes dramatic and usually instantaneous onset of severe headache.

FAINTS AND FITS

Transient loss of consciousness may have a neurological cause but cardiac arrhythmias and metabolic diseases are other possible explanations. The following should be considered.

Syncope due to a simple faint is the most common cause of loss of consciousness. The episode is usually very brief and is often preceded by pallor, sweating, nausea and dizziness. If the degree of cerebral hypoperfusion is severe, there may be a few clonic jerks or a brief tonic spasm ('convulsive syncope').

Epilepsy: abrupt loss of consciousness which may be preceded by an aura — an abnormal sensation (e.g., an hallucination involving one of the senses or altered cognition such as a sense of deja vu). Bystanders may have observed tonic (sustained contraction of the muscles for 15 to 20 seconds) and clonic (violent rhythmical) movements. However, cerebral hypoxia of any cause, (e.g., from severe bradycardia) can cause these movements. The patient who has had a major seizure may sleep for a period after the episode and may wake to find he or she has bitten the tongue and been incontinent.

Transient ischaemic attacks affecting the brainstem. These may rarely cause loss of consciousness without warning.

Hypoglycaemia (usually in diabetic patients on insulin or taking oral hypoglycaemic drugs). These patients may feel anxious, sweaty and notice a fast heart rate before unconsciousness occurs — these are autonomic responses to hypoglycaemia.

Hysteria may cause bizarre attacks of apparent loss of consciousness.

VERTIGO AND DIZZINESS

In true **vertigo**, there is actually a sense of motion. The world seems to turn around. This can be caused by vestibular disease (such as acute labyrinthitis, benign positional vertigo or Ménière's disease) or brainstem disease (such as that caused by alcohol, anticonvulsants, multiple sclerosis, vascular lesions or tumour).

Dizziness can be a feeling of impending unconsciousness or merely of momentary unsteadiness.

VISUAL DISTURBANCES AND DEAFNESS

Ask about; double vision (diplopia), blurred vision, loss of vision (amblyopia) and light intolerance (photophobia). Ask also about loss of hearing in one or both ears, and about ringing in the ears (tinnitus).

DISTURBANCES OF GAIT

Many neurological conditions can make walking difficult. Cerebellar disease makes walking unsteady and uncertain. Hemiplegia makes walking difficult because of an increase in tone and loss of power in the affected leg. A peripheral neuropathy or spinal cord disease may alter position sense in the legs. Walking may also be abnormal when orthopaedic disease affects the lower limbs or spine. Parkinson's disease causes a characteristic shuffling gait. Hysteria can also present with a bizarrely abnormal gait.

DISTURBED SENSATION OR WEAKNESS IN THE LIMBS

Pins and needles in the hands or feet more often indicate nerve entrapment or a peripheral neuropathy but can result from sensory pathway involvement at any level.

Weakness may be due to cerebral, spinal cord (including anterior horn cell), nerve root, peripheral nerve, neuromuscular junction or muscle disease. Distinguishing between an upper and lower motor neurone lesion is important (Table 5.4).

TREMOR AND INVOLUNTARY MOVEMENTS

Tremors are fine involuntary repetitive movements. Action tremors are worse when a voluntary movement is attempted. These include an enhanced physiological tremor, as may occur in essential tremors, anxiety and thyrotoxicosis. Intention (or target seeking) tremor becomes worse as the limb gets closer to an object reached for and is due to cerebellar disease. **Parkinson's disease** may present with a resting tremor while in **chorea** there are irregular jerky movements.

PAST HEALTH

Inquire about a past history of meningitis or encephalitis, head or spinal injuries, epilepsy, or risk factors for HIV infection or syphilis which may have nervous system involvement. Anticonvulsant drugs, the contraceptive pill, antihypertensive agents, anti-Parkinsonian drugs, steroids, anticoagulants and antiplatelet agents may all be used for neurological conditions or have neurological effects and need to be documented. Ask about risk factors

TABLE 5.1 Neurological History

Presenting Symptoms
Headache
Facial pain
Back or neck pain
Fits, faints or funny turns
Dizziness or vertigo
Disturbances of vision, hearing or smell
Disturbances of gait
Loss of or disturbed sensation, or weakness in a limb(s)
Disturbances of sphincter control (bladder, bowels)
Involuntary movements or tremor
Speech and swallowing disturbance
Altered cognition

Risk Factors for Cerebrovascular Disease
Hypertension
Smoking
Diabetes mellitus
Hyperlipidaemia
Atrial fibrillation, bacterial endocarditis, myocardial
    infarction (emboli), valvular heart disease
Haematological disease
Family history of stroke

that may predispose to the development of cerebrovascular disease (Table 5.1).

SOCIAL HISTORY

As smoking predisposes to cerebrovascular disease, the smoking history is relevant. It is also useful to ask about occupation and exposure to toxins (e.g., heavy metals). Alcohol can also result in a number of neurological diseases such as cerebellar degeneration and peripheral neuropathy.

TABLE 5.2 The Mini-Mental State Examination

	Score	Max
Orientation		
'What is the (year) (season) (date) (day) (month)?'		
Ask for the date, then specifically inquire about parts omitted (e.g., season).	☐	5
Score 1 point for each correct answer.		
'Where are we (country) (state) (town) (hospital) (ward)?'		
Ask in turn for each place.	☐	5
Score 1 point for each correct answer.		

Registration

'May I test your memory?'
Repeat three objects (e.g., pen, watch, book).

Score 1 point for each correct answer. ☐ 3
Then repeat until the patient learns all three.

Count trials and record (up to six).

Attention and Calculation

'Count backwards from 100 by sevens' (Serial 7s).
One point for each answer, up to five ☐ 5
(93, 86, 79, 72, 65)

or

Spell 'world' backwards.
Score 1 point for each letter in correct order.

Recall

Ask the patient to recall the three objects in 'registration', above.
Score 1 point for each correct answer. ☐ 3

TABLE 5.2 Continued

Language

Ask the patient to name two objects shown (e.g., pen and watch). Score 0–2 points.	☐	2
'Repeat the following: "No ifs, ands or buts".' Score 1 point.	☐	1
Ask the patient to follow a three-stage command: e.g., 'Take this paper in your right hand, fold it in half and put it on the table.' Score 1 point for each step.	☐	3
Read and obey the folowing: CLOSE YOUR EYES. Score 1 point.	☐	1
WRITE A SENTENCE. Do not dictate — must be sensible, but punctuation and grammar not essential. Score 1 point.	☐	1
'Copy this design.'	☐	1

All ten angles must be present, and the
two must intersect.
Score 1 point

TOTAL	☐	30

Assess patient's level of consciousness along a continuum

Alert	Drowsy	Stuporous	Coma

Scores of 21 to 29 indicate mild cognitive impairment.
Scores below 20 indicate more severe cognitive
impairment, and are highly likely to be due to dementia,
especially if obtained on repeated examinations.

FAMILY HISTORY

Any history of neurological or mental disease should be documented.

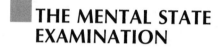 THE MENTAL STATE EXAMINATION

Any patient who has a history of confusion, or is suspected of having dementia or a major psychiatric illness should have a mental state examination performed. A rapid way of testing for orientation, memory and attention is to have the patient complete a mini-mental state examination (Table 5.2). Even gross disturbances of these functions may not be obvious unless they are formally tested.

NEUROLOGICAL EXAMINATION TECHNIQUE

The neurological examination is complicated but rewarding. Adequate interpretation of neurological signs requires an understanding of basic neuroanatomy. The following components must be systematically assessed.

General

This includes examination for the level of consciousness, the presence of neck stiffness and the assessment of the higher centres and speech.

The Cranial Nerves

Examine the cranial nerves II (including the fundi) to XII. The first (olfactory) nerve is often omitted.

The Upper Limbs

Motor system: inspection, tone, power, reflexes and coordination. **Sensory system pain:** (pin prick) sensation, light touch, proprioception (position sense) and vibration sense.

The Lower Limbs

As for the upper limbs (motor and sensory systems), but including assessment of walking (gait).

The Skull and Spine

Assess for local disease if relevant.

The Carotid Arteries

Auscultate both sides for bruits.

NECK STIFFNESS AND KERNIG'S SIGN

This examination is absolutely essential for any febrile or acutely ill patient. The examiner slips one hand under the patient's head and attempts gently to flex the head so that the patient's chin touches the chest (Figure 5.1). Resistance due to painful spasm of the extensor muscles of the neck will occur if the meninges are inflamed.

The examiner should next flex the hip and then attempt to straighten the patient's knee — **Kernig's sign** (Figure 5.2). Painful spasm of the hamstrings will occur if there is inflammation around the lumbar spinal roots.

HANDEDNESS, ORIENTATION SPEECH AND HIGHER CENTRES

Ask the patient if he or she is right or left handed (to help determine the likely dominant hemisphere).

As a screening assessment, ask for the patient's name, present location and the date. This tests orientation in **person**,

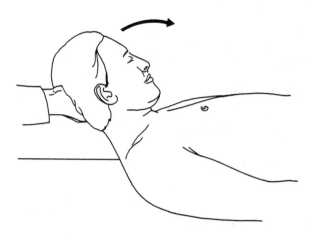

FIGURE 5.1 Testing for neck stiffness.

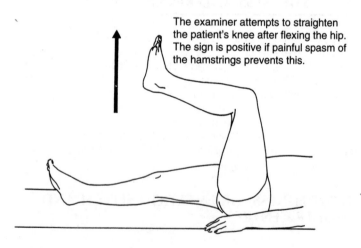

The examiner attempts to straighten the patient's knee after flexing the hip. The sign is positive if painful spasm of the hamstrings prevents this.

FIGURE 5.2 Kernig's Sign.

place and **time**. These tests are part of the mini-mental state examination.

Next ask the patient to name an object pointed at and have him or her point to a named object in the room. This screens for dysphasia (**receptive dysphasia** — inability to understand speech; **expressive dysphasia** — inability to answer appropriately; **nominal dysphasia** — inability to name objects; or **conductive aphasia** — inability to repeat speech). See Table 5.3.

Dysarthria is a problem with the mechanical production of speech. Ask the patient to say 'West Register Street' or 'British Constitution'. This is a test for cerebellar dysfunction and its effect on speech. Cerebellar disease causes slurring and staccato speech.

TABLE 5.3 Examination of a Patient with Dysphasia

Fluent Speech (Receptive, Conductive or Nominal Aphasia, Usually)

1. Name objects. Patients with nominal, conductive or receptive aphasia will name objects poorly.

2. Repetition. Conductive and receptive aphasic patients have difficulty repeating.

3. Comprehension. Only receptive aphasic patients cannot follow commands (verbal or written).

4. Reading aloud. Conductive and receptive aphasic patients may have difficulty (dyslexia).

Non-fluent Speech (Expressive Aphasia, Usually)

1. Naming of objects. This is poor but may be better than spontaneous speech.

TABLE 5.3   Continued

2. Repetition. May be possible with great effort. Phrase repetition (e.g., 'no ifs, ands or buts') is poor.

3. Comprehension often mildly impaired despite popular belief but written and verbal commands are followed.

4. Reading. Patients may have dyslexia.

5. Writing. Dysgraphia may be present.

6. Look for hemiparesis. The arm is more affected than the leg.

CRANIAL NERVES

The patient should be sat over the edge of the bed.

Begin by general inspection of the head and neck. Look for **craniotomy** scars which suggest previous surgery which has required opening of the skull.

The cranial nerves are then examined in roughly the order of their number. The use of a systematic approach is the only way to be sure nothing important is left out.

The First (Olfactory) Nerve

Testing is not performed routinely but is required if there is suspected loss of smell (anosmia). Each nostril is tested separately using non-pungent substances in a series of sample bottles. The patient sniffs these delicately and should be able to identify common smells such as coffee and vanilla.

The Second (Optic) Nerve (see also Chapter 6)

Always test **visual acuity** with the patient wearing his or her spectacles. Each eye is tested separately, while the other is covered with a small card. The patient is asked to read letters on a chart. The standard chart is read reflected in a mirror from 3 metres away (effectively 6 metres). Ability to read the letters normally visible at this distance is called 6/6 vision. Ability only to read larger letters normally visible at 60 metres is called 6/60 vision. Patients with poor visual acuity may only be able to distinguish hand movements or light and dark.

Examine the **visual fields**. One method is by confrontation using a red-topped hat pin. In this examination the patient's field of vision is compared with the examiner's (Figure 5.3). The examiner's head should be level with the patient's head. Each eye is tested separately. The pin is brought into the visual field of the examiner and patient, and should become visible to each at the same point. The pin should be brought into each quadrant diagonally.

If visual acuity is poor, the fields are mapped using the fingers instead of the pin. The patient is asked to say when the examiner's first and second fingers become visible as they are brought into the quadrants of the visual fields.

Look into the fundi (page 169).

The Third (Oculomotor), Fourth (Trochlear) and Sixth (Abducens) Nerves

These nerves control eye movements, the upper eyelid and pupil size, and are usually tested together. Look at the **pupils**, noting the shape, relative sizes and any associated **ptosis**. If one or both pupils are small this is called miosis and causes include eye drops for glaucoma, narcotics, Horner's Syndrome (interruption of the sympathetic innervation of the eye which also causes ptosis of the eyelid), or a pontine brain haemorrhage (and rarely syphilis — the Argyll-Robertson pupil).

Enlargement of the pupils is called mydriasis. Causes include a third nerve palsy (unilateral) and instillation of mydriatic eye drops. Other causes include Adie's pupil, trauma and iritis with synechiae. Unequal pupils may be physiological and this condition is called essential anisocoria.

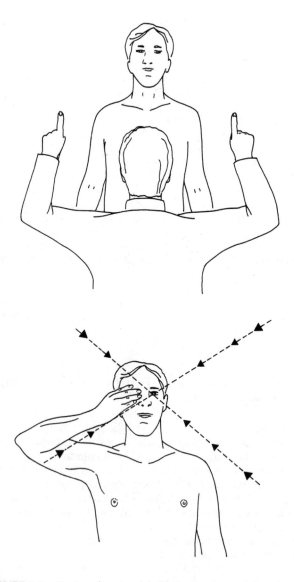

FIGURE 5.3 Testing the visual fields by confrontation.

Use a pocket torch and shine the light from the side to gauge the **reaction of the pupils to light**. Assess quickly both the normal **direct** (constriction of the illuminated pupil) and normal **consensual** (constriction of the other pupil) responses. **Both** pupils should contract briskly and equally when a light is shone into **one**.

Test **accommodation** (the constriction of the pupils that occurs when the eyes focus on a near object) by asking the patient to look into the distance and then at an object (e.g., a hat pin or a pen) placed about 20 cm from the nose.

Assess eye movements with both eyes first, getting the patient to follow the pin or finger laterally right and left, then up and down (in an H pattern). Look for failure of movement (remember that the lateral rectus, supplied by the sixth nerve, only moves the eye horizontally outwards. See Figure 6.1). Ask about **diplopia** (double vision) and in which direction of gaze the diplopia is most pronounced. Diplopia may be due to weakness of one or more of the ocular muscles. The separation of the images is greatest in the direction in which the affected muscle has its dominant effect.

Look for **nystagmus**. This is really an involuntary rhythmic oscillation of the ocular muscles back and forth. It may be pendular where the oscillations of the eye occur centrally and are equal in each direction. This usually indicates a problem with fixation. **Phasic** (jerky) **nystagmus** involves a slow drifting movement and a rapid correcting movement. The direction of the nystagmus is defined as the direction of the fast phase. Phasic nystagmus is a sign of cerebellar, brainstem or vestibular disease. Fine phasic nystagmus is normal at the extremes of gaze so testing should involve asking the patient to follow the examiner's finger so that each eye is abducted about 30° in turn.

Remember the characteristic signs of palsies of the third, fourth and fifth nerves.

THIRD NERVE

Ipsilateral (same side as the lesion) mydriasis which is unreactive to light or accommodation, complete ptosis and divergent strabismus (the eye is deviated down and out).

FOURTH NERVE

Inability to turn the eye **down and in**.

SIXTH NERVE

Failure of lateral movement, with diploplia most pronounced on looking laterally.

The Fifth (Trigeminal) Nerve

Test the **corneal reflexes** gently using a wisp of cotton wool to touch the cornea and ask the patient if the touch can be felt. Normally the eyelids should **both** shut briskly. The sensory component of this reflex is the fifth nerve and the motor component is the seventh nerve.

Test facial sensation in the three divisions: ophthalmic, maxillary and mandibular (Figure 5.4).

Test **pain** (pin prick) sensation with the pin in each area. Start on one side of the forehead and move to the other side, pressing the pin into the skin and asking the patient to tell you what he or she feels (sharp is normal!); don't press hard enough to draw blood. Map any area of sensory loss. If areas of reduced sensation (dull) are found, map them by moving the pin until normal sensation is again present (sharp) (see page 156).

Test **light touch** by touching but not stroking the skin with a piece of cotton wool.

Note the presence of **sensory dissociation** (usually loss of pain and temperature sensation and preservation of light touch). This is rare but occurs typically in syringobulbia, where enlargement of the central canal of the brainstem and upper spinal cord interrupts crossing pain and temperature fibres first.

Examine the **motor** division of the fifth nerve by asking the patient to **clench** the teeth while you feel the masseter muscles. Then get the patient to **open the mouth** while you attempt to **force it closed**; this is not possible if the pterygoid muscles are working. A unilateral lesion causes the jaw to deviate towards the weak (**affected**) side because the normal muscle's action is unopposed.

Test the **jaw jerk** by tapping the reflex hammer on your own thumb placed on the chin of the patient. This is present in normal people but is exaggerated, with brisk bilateral contraction of the masseter muscles, in cases of **pseudobulbar palsy** (bilateral upper motor neurone lesions also affecting IX, X and XII). (See page 145 and Table 5.4).

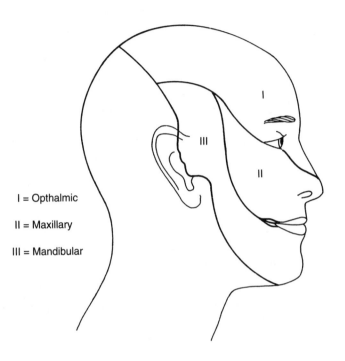

I = Opthalmic

II = Maxillary

III = Mandibular

FIGURE 5.4 The divisions of the trigeminal nerve.

The Seventh (Facial) Nerve

Test the muscles of **facial expression**. Ask the patient to look up and wrinkle the forehead. Look for loss of wrinkling and feel the muscle strength by pushing down on each side. This is preserved in upper motor neurone lesions because of **bilateral** cortical representation of these muscles.

Next ask the patient to shut the eyes tightly and compare the two sides. Both upper and lower facial weakness leads to incomplete closure of the eye on the same side but a lower motor neurone lesion has a more pronounced effect. Tell the patient to grin and compare the nasolabial grooves.

TABLE 5.4 Upper and Lower Motor Neurone Lesions

Signs of Upper Motor Neurone Lesions

1. Weakness is present which in the lower limb is more marked in the flexor and abductor muscles. In the upper limb, weakness is more marked in the abductors and extensors. There is very little muscle wasting (unless from disuse).

2. Spasticity: increased tone is present (may be clasp-knife — initial resistance which gives way suddenly) and often associated with clonus.

3. The reflexes are increased except for the superficial reflexes (e.g., abdominal) which are absent.

4. There is an extensor (Babinski) plantar response (upgoing toe).

Signs of Lower Motor Neurone Lesions

1. Weakness may be more obvious distally than proximally, and the flexor and extensor muscles are equally involved. Wasting is a prominent feature.

2. Tone is reduced.

3. The reflexes are reduced and the plantar response is normal or absent.

4. Fasciculation may be present.

The Eighth (Acoustic) Nerve

Quantitative hearing assessment is not possible without special equipment but useful qualitative information can be obtained at the bedside. Whisper softly a number 60 cm away from each ear whilst the other is distracted by movement of the examiner's finger in the auditory canal. It takes practice to get an idea of what loudness a whisper is normally audible.

If there is deafness, perform **Rinne's** and **Weber's** tests and examine the external auditory canals and the eardrums (Chapter 6).

The Ninth (Glossopharyngeal) and Tenth (Vagus) Nerves

Look at the palate and note any **uvular displacement**. Ask the patient to say 'ah' and look for symmetrical movement of the soft palate. With a unilateral lesion of the tenth nerve the uvula is drawn towards the unaffected (normal) side.

It may be unwise to test even gently for a **gag** reflex (the **ninth** nerve is the sensory component and the **tenth** nerve the motor component). A spatula is touched onto each side of the soft palate in turn. The normal response is gagging with contraction of the palate on both sides or even vomiting. It is probably preferable to touch the pharynx on each side and ask if the touch can be felt and seems the same on each side. The efferent limb of this reflex has been tested when the patient said 'ah'. Ask the patient to speak to assess **hoarseness**, and to cough and swallow. A 'bovine' or hollow cough suggests bilateral recurrent laryngeal nerve lesions.

The Twelfth (Hypoglossal) Nerve

While examining the mouth inspect the tongue for wasting and **fasciculation** (random flickering movements of small muscle groups) which is characteristic of a lower motor neurone lesion (page 151).

Next ask the patient to protrude the tongue. With a unilateral lesion the tongue deviates towards the weaker (affected) side.

The Eleventh (Accessory) Nerve

Ask the patient to shrug the shoulders and feel the trapezius as you push the shoulders down. Then ask the patient to turn the head against resistance and also feel the bulk of the sternomastoid. The normal muscle turns the head to the opposite side. Nerve palsy (a lower motor neurone lesion) causes weak contraction of the sternomastoid ipsilateral to the lesion (i.e. weakness of head turning to the opposite side). An upper motor neurone lesion may cause weakness of contralateral head version because of ipsilateral sternomastoid weakness.

UPPER LIMBS

Ask the patient to sit over the side of the bed facing you. **Look** for abnormal movements.

1. **Tremor.** A tremor is rhythmical oscillation around a joint due to contraction and relaxation of muscles or alternating contraction and relaxation in opposing muscle groups. A normal (**static** or **action**) fine (>10 cycles/second) tremor is present when muscles attempt to maintain a stationary position against gravity (physiological tremor). This is exaggerated with anxiety, alcoholism and thyrotoxicosis and in patients with a familial tremor. A coarse 4 to 7 cycles per second resting tremor occurs in Parkinson's disease. There is repetitive flexion and contraction of the fingers and abduction and adduction of the thumb (pill rolling tremor) at rest.

2. **Irregular movements. Choreiform** movements are involuntary jerky repetitive movements that may appear to be semi-purposeful; they occur in extra-pyramidal disease. Flapping of the tongue (rapid protrusion and retraction with flapping of the tip) is commonly associated. **Athetosis** is a slow writhing movement. The dramatic involuntary swinging movements that characterise **hemiballismus** are rare. **Myoclonic jerks** on the other hand are involuntary sudden shock-like muscle contractions that are relatively common.

3. **Pseudoathetosis** (small writhing movements, especially of the fingers) occurs because of proprioceptive loss.

Motor System

Examine the motor system systematically every time.

Inspect first for **wasting** (both proximal and distal) and **fasciculations**. Don't forget to include the shoulder girdle in your inspection.

Ask the patient to hold both hands out with the arms extended and to close the eyes. **Look** for drifting of one or both arms which can only be due to upper motor neurone weakness, a cerebellar lesion or proprioceptive loss.

Feel the muscle bulk and note any muscle tenderness.

Remember the difference between upper and lower motor neurone lesions. A lesion which interrupts the neural pathway above the anterior horn cell in the spinal cord is called an **upper motor neurone lesion**. Examples include lesions of the cerebral cortex, internal capsule, brainstem or upper spinal cord. These are associated with increased tone (spasticity) in the affected muscle groups. The reflexes are exaggerated, clonus (see page 151) may be present but muscle wasting and fasciculations are absent. **Lower motor neurone** lesions result in reduced tone and reflexes, muscle wasting and sometimes fasciculations (Table 5.4).

Test tone at the wrists and elbows by moving the joints passively at varying velocities. Flex and extend the patient's wrists and elbows after asking him or her to relax and not help you. It takes some practice to become familiar with normal muscle tone. Increased tone is easier to detect than decreased tone. Changes in tone are also easier to detect if they are unilateral.

Assess power (Figure 5.5) at the shoulders, elbows, wrists and fingers. Remember that right handed people are slightly stronger on the right side. Power is graded as follows:

1. — complete paralysis
2. — a flicker of contraction
3. — movement is possible where gravity is excluded
4. — movement is possible against gravity but not if any further resistance is added
5. — movement is possible against gravity and some resistance
6. — normal power.

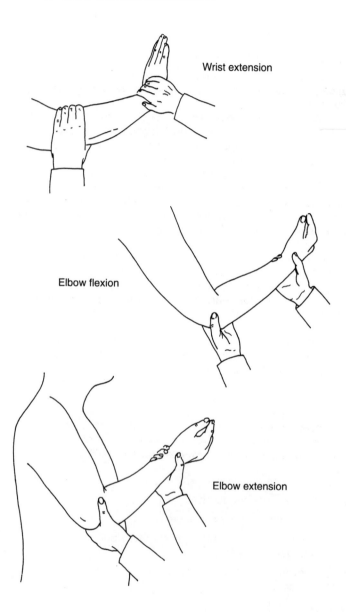

Wrist extension

Elbow flexion

Elbow extension

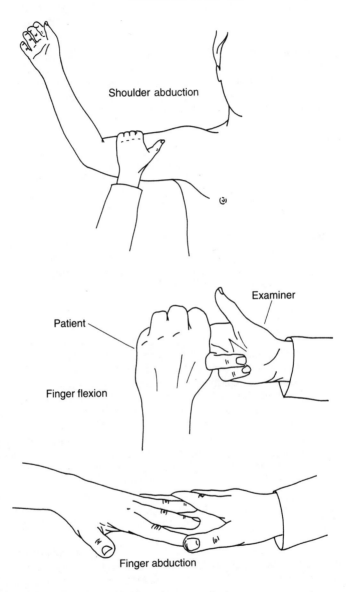

FIGURE 5.5 Testing power in the upper limbs.

SHOULDER

Abduction (C5, C6): the patient should abduct the arms with the elbows flexed and resist the examiner's attempt to push them down. **Adduction** (C6, C7, C8): the patient should adduct the arms with the elbows flexed and not allow the examiner to separate them.

ELBOW

Flexion (C5, C6): the patient should bend the elbow and pull so as not to let the examiner straighten it out. **Extension** (C7): the patient should bend the elbow and push so as not to let the examiner bend it.

WRIST

Flexion (C6, C7, C8): the patient should bend the wrist and not allow the examiner to straighten it. **Extension** (C7, C8): the patient should extend the wrist and not allow the examiner to bend it.

FINGERS

Extension (C7, C8): the patient should straighten the fingers and not allow the examiner to push them down (push with the side of your hand across the patient's metacarpophalangeal joints).

Flexion (C7, C8): the patient squeezes two of the examiner's fingers. **Abduction** (C8, T1): the patient should spread out the fingers and not allow the examiner to push them together.

If the patient has a **claw hand** (fixed contraction of the fingers) testing for an **ulnar** or **median** nerve lesion is necessary. There will be wasting of the small muscles of the hand with deep gutters between the long extensor tendons and hypothenar eminence (ulnar nerve lesion) or thenar eminence (median nerve lesion).

When the patient grasps a piece of paper between the thumb and the lateral aspect of the forefinger the thumb flexes if an ulnar lesion has caused loss of the adductor of the thumb (Froment's sign).

Ask the patient to place the hand flat, with the palm upwards and then ask him or her to lift the thumb vertically against resistance or to lift the thumb vertically to touch the examiner's pen (pen touching test for loss of abductor pollicis brevis — median nerve; Figure 5.6).

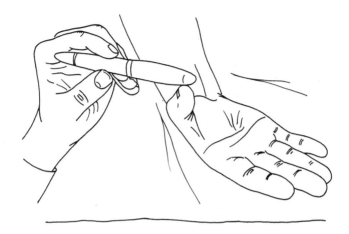

FIGURE 5.6   The pen touching test for loss of abductor pollicis brevis (median nerve).

Reflexes

Examine the reflexes (Figure 5.7) routinely at the elbow and wrist.

Remember that the **reflex arc** consists of afferent and efferent pathways. The afferent pathway is stimulated when a tendon is stretched (e.g., after being struck by a reflex hammer). The afferent pathway synapses in the spinal cord with a motor neurone which fires, stimulating the efferent pathway, and causes contraction of the opposing muscle to release the stretch on the tendon. Interruption of the efferent or afferent limb of the reflex arc prevents contraction and the reflex is absent. Interruption of pathways in the spinal cord above the level of the motor neurone (upper motor neurone lesion) releases this from inhibition and causes exaggerated reflexes (Table 5.4). Reflexes may be normal, increased, decreased, absent or delayed (contraction is brisk but return is slow — typical of hypothyroidism).

Clonus is rhythmical contraction of the muscle that can continue as long as tension is maintained on the tendon.

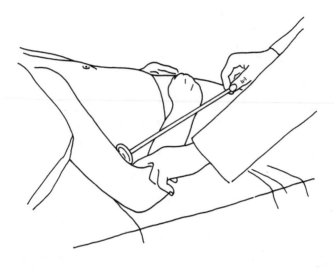

The biceps jerk

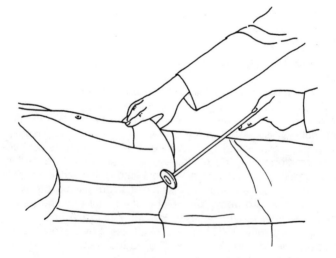

The triceps jerk

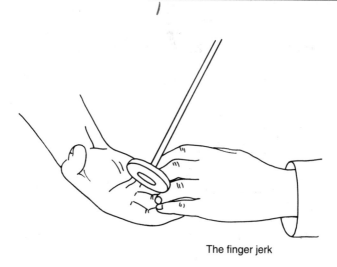

The finger jerk

FIGURE 5.7 The biceps and triceps and finger jerks.

An idea of the range of normal reflexes can only be obtained by practice. Always compare right with left. Upper limb tendon reflexes are sometimes difficult to elicit in youth.

Biceps (C5, C6): the examiner's left forefinger is placed over the biceps tendon and the patellar hammer allowed to fall on to it. There is normally a brisk (but not too brisk) contraction of the biceps muscle.

Triceps (C7, C8): the examiner supports one of the patient's elbows with one hand and taps over the triceps tendon with the hammer. There is normally triceps contraction and extension of the forearm.

Brachioradialis (C5, C6): the examiner places a few fingers over the lower end of the radius and strikes them. Contraction of the brachioradialis causes flexion of the elbow.

Finger (C8, T1): the examiner interlocks his or her hand with the patient's while the patient's hand is resting palm upwards; the tendon hammer is used to strike the examiner's hand. Normally, there is slight flexion of all fingers and of the interphalangeal joint of the thumb.

In patients with suspected upper motor neurone disease, **Hoffman's reflex** can also be elicited: the terminal part of the patient's middle finger is flicked downwards between the examiner's thumb and finger; it is abnormal if the thumb flexes and adducts while the other fingers flex. The presence of this reflex indicates hyper-reflexia but is *not* pathognomonic of an upper motor neurone disease.

The reflexes can be recorded as:

0 (absent)

+ (reduced)

++ (normal)

+++ (increased)

+++ (exaggerated and with clonus).

Assess Coordination (Cerebellar Function)

First apply **finger-nose testing**. The patient is asked to touch the tip of the examiner's forefinger with his or her own forefinger and with the arm extended and then to touch his or her own nose (Figure 5.8). The movements are alternated rapidly. Cerebellar disease will cause the patient's finger to oscillate and overshoot. It

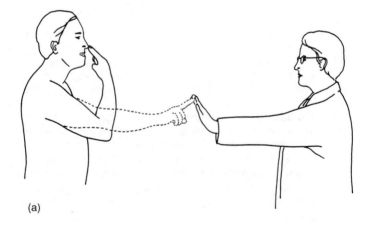

(a)

(b)

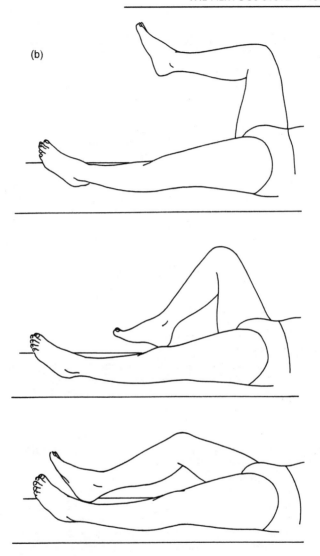

FIGURE 5.8 The cerebellar examination. (a) finger-nose test,
(b) heel-shin test.

is best to keep the target finger still to obtain a better idea of muscle control.

Examine for **dysdiadochokinesis**, the inability to perform rapidly alternating movements such as supinating and pronating the wrists repeatedly (this action appears clumsy in the presence of cerebellar disease).

Next look for **rebound**. The patient attempts to lift the arm against resistance; when this is released suddenly the arm rebounds upwards in cerebellar disease.

Remember motor weakness can be due to an **upper motor neurone** lesion (hyper-reflexia with absence of wasting), a **lower motor neurone** lesion (wasting due to denervation, absent reflexes), **neuromuscular transmission disorders** (fatigue on repeated muscle use) or a **myopathy**, (muscle disease: usually with wasting but with variable reflexes). If there is evidence of a lower motor neurone lesion, consider anterior horn cell, nerve root or brachial plexus lesions, peripheral nerve lesions or a motor peripheral neuropathy.

Sensory System

Examine the **sensory system** after motor testing, because this can be time-consuming.

First test the **spinothalamic pathway (pain and temperature)**. Demonstrate to the patient the sharpness of a new pin on the anterior chest wall or forehead. Do not use an injection needle. These are too sharp and can draw blood. Then ask the patient to close the eyes and tell you if the sensation is sharp or dull. Start proximally and test pin prick in each dermatome (Figure 5.9). As you are assessing, try to fit any sensory loss into **dermatomal** — loss fits into the pattern of one or more dermatomes (cord or nerve root lesion), **peripheral nerve** (pattern specific for the nerve affected e.g., median or ulna nerve), peripheral neuropathy (affected area is in the shape of a **glove**) or **hemisensory** — loss involves one side (cortical or cord) distribution. Always compare proximal with distal, side with side and look for a sensory level. Tap the pin a number of times in each place to ensure reproducibility.

Next test the **posterior column pathway (vibration and proprioception)**. Use a 128 Hz tuning fork to assess **vibration** sense. Place the vibrating fork on a distal interphalangeal joint when the patient has the eyes closed and ask if the vibrations can

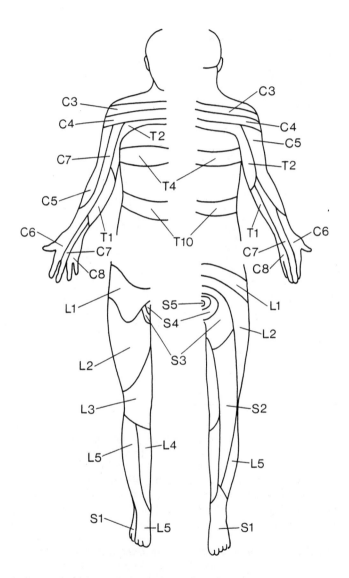

FIGURE 5.9 The dermatomes of the limbs.

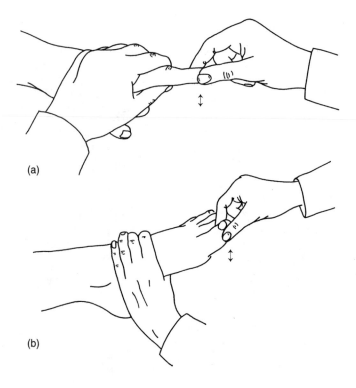

FIGURE 5.10 Testing proprioception; (a) finger, (b) toe.

be felt. If so, ask the patient to tell you when the vibration ceases and then, after a short wait, stop the fork vibrating. If the patient has deficient sensation, test at the wrist, then elbow, then at the shoulder to determine the level of the sensory loss.

Examine **proprioception** first with the distal interphalangeal joint of the index finger (Figure 5.10). When the patient has the eyes open grasp the distal phalanx from the sides and move it up and down to demonstrate, then ask the patient to close the eyes; repeat the manoeuvre. Normally, movement through even a few degrees is detectable, and the patient can tell if it is up or down. If there is an abnormality, proceed to test the wrist and elbows similarly to determine the level of the lesion.

Test **light touch** with cotton wool. Touch the skin lightly in each dermatome.

Test for **cortical sensory abnormalities**, if a cortical lesion is suspected after the initial examination. Parietal lobe lesions may cause **sensory inattention**. Here sensation is normal when one side at a time is tested but absent on the opposite side to the lesion if both sides are tested together. The patient shuts the eyes and both hands are touched. The stimulus is felt only on the normal side. **Astereognosis** also occurs with parietal lesions. This is inability to recognise an object placed in the patient's hand.

LOWER LIMBS

Gait

Test the stance and gait first if possible (Figure 5.11).

Ask the patient to walk normally for a short distance and then to turn around quickly and come back. Then ask him or her to walk heel to toe (a test of cerebellar function which has been used by the police to test for alcohol intoxication in less sophisticated times), then to walk on the toes (impossible with an S1 or tibial nerve lesion) and finally on the heels (impossible with an L4-5 or peroneal nerve lesion).

Ask the patient to stand with the feet together first with the eyes open and then with them closed. Increased swaying when the eyes are open suggests cerebellar disease. If this only occurs when the eyes are closed (**Romberg's sign**) it suggests proprioceptive loss.

Motor System

Put the patient in bed with the legs entirely exposed. Place a towel over the groin — note whether a urinary catheter is present.

Look for **muscle wasting** and **fasciculations**. Note any tremor.

Feel the **muscle bulk** of the **quadriceps** and run your hand up each shin, feeling for wasting of the **anterior tibial** muscles.

Test tone at the knees and ankles. The patient lies supine and is asked to relax and not oppose or assist movement of the limbs by the examiner. The examiner's hand is placed under the patient's knee and the knee lifted quickly so that it flexes. The foot is

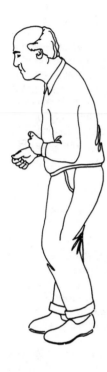

Parkinsonian gait – stooped posture, small hurried shuffling steps (festination).

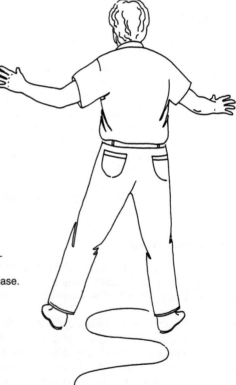

A wide-based staggering gait – cerebellar or labyrinthine disease.

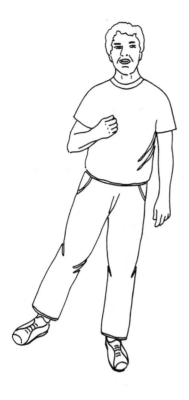

Right hemiplegic –
the right leg
swings outwards
in an arc.

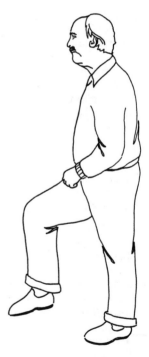

High stepping
gait – peripheral
neuropathy.

FIGURE 5.11 Gait disturbances.

then grasped by the examiner and flexed and extended repeatedly. With practice, normal and abnormal muscle resistance to these movements will be appreciated.

Test **clonus** at this time. Push the lower end of the quadriceps sharply down towards the knee. Sustained rhythmical contractions of the quadriceps indicate an upper motor neurone lesion. Also test the ankle by sharply dorsiflexing the foot with the knee bent and the thigh externally rotated; look for clonus of the calf muscles.

Assess power next at the hips, knees and ankles. This should again be graded from 0 to 5.

HIP

Flexion (L2, L3 innervation): ask the patient to lift up the straight leg and not to let you push it down (having placed your hand above the knee).

Extension (S1): ask the patient to keep the leg down and not to let you pull it up from underneath the calf or ankle.

Abduction (L5): ask the patient to abduct the leg and not to let you push it in.

Adduction (L2, L3): ask the patient to keep the leg adducted and not to let you push it out.

KNEE

Flexion (L5, S1): ask the patient to bend the knee and not to let you straighten it.

Extension (L3, L4): with the knee slightly bent, ask the patient to straighten the knee and not to let you bend it.

ANKLE

Plantar flexion (S1, S2): ask the patient to push the foot down and not to let you push it up.

Dorsiflexion (L4, L5): ask the patient to bring the foot up and not to let you push it down.

Eversion (L5): ask the patient to evert the foot against resistance.

Inversion (L5, S1): with the foot in complete plantar flexion, ask the patient to invert the foot against resistance.

Reflexes

Examine the reflexes (Figure 5.12)

KNEE (L3, L4)

Allow the patellar hammer to fall elegantly onto the infrapatellar tendon while the patient's knee is supported by the examiner's arm. Watch for contraction of the quadriceps.

ANKLE (S1, S2)

The patient's foot is in the mid-position at the ankle, the knee is bent and the thigh is externally rotated on the bed. The patellar hammer is allowed to fall on to the patellar tendon. Plantar flexion of the foot will normally occur.

PLANTAR RESPONSE (L5, S1, S2)

A key or similar object is run slowly along the lateral aspect of the patient's sole. The normal response is flexion of the great toe. Upper motor neurone lesions result in extension of the great toe and fanning of the other toes. This is described as an upgoing plantar response or a positive **Babinski's sign**.

Test Coordination

Perform the **heel-shin** test (the patient runs the heel of one foot up and down the shin of the other leg as rapidly and accurately as possible, while the examiner looks for wobbling (Figure 5.8, pages 154–5); **toe-finger** test (the patient brings the toe up to touch the examiner's forefinger with the knee bent, while the examiner looks for tremor and overshooting); and **tapping of the feet** (the patient taps the sole of the foot on the examiner's hand, while the examiner looks for clumsy or slow movements — **dysdiadochokinesis**).

Examine the Sensory System

Test pain (pinprick), then **vibration and proprioception**, and then **light touch** (as described for the upper limbs in each dermatome). (See Figure 5.9) If there is a peripheral sensory loss, attempt to establish the sensory level on the trunk.

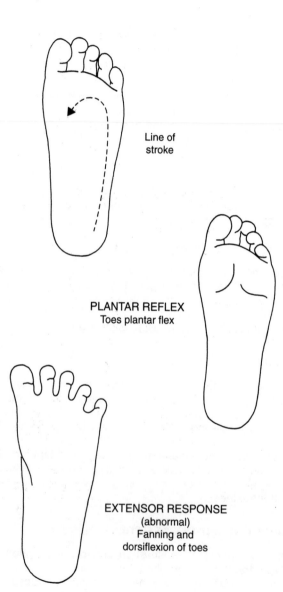

Line of
stroke

PLANTAR REFLEX
Toes plantar flex

EXTENSOR RESPONSE
(abnormal)
Fanning and
dorsiflexion of toes

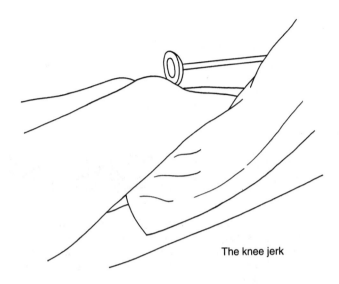

The knee jerk

FIGURE 5.12 The knee and plantar reflexes.

Test the abdominal reflexes. The skin of the lower abdominal wall is stroked with a sharpish object such as a key, first on one side and then on the other. Brisk contraction of the underlying muscles normally occurs. Test the upper and lower quadrants on both sides. Absent reflexes may be a result of an upper motor neurone lesion, of lax abdominal muscles or of previous surgery that has cut the superficial abdominal nerves.

Examine sensation in the **saddle region** (perineum and medial aspects of the upper thighs) region and test the **anal reflex** (S2, S3, S4); there is normally contraction of the external sphincter in response to scratching of the perianal skin.

Examine the back. Look for deformity, scars and neuro-fibromas. Palpate for tenderness over the vertebral bodies and auscultate for bruits. Any of these may indicate spinal cord abnormalities.

Perform the straight leg raising test. Lie the patient flat and slowly flex the hip while keeping the knee fully extended. Tell the patient to advise you as soon as there is pain and where it occurs (a disc compression of the lumbar or sacral roots will limit leg raising because of pain in the ipsilateral leg that will be increased by foot dorsiflexion). With more severe nerve root irritation the pain will be felt in the other lower limb as well (crossed straight leg raising sign). Test the upper lumbar roots by lying the patient prone and extending the hip (while the knee is flexed to 90°) see page 135.

THE NEUROLOGICAL EXAMINATION — HINTS

1. A careful neurological history should direct the neurological examination to the most relevant areas. Symptoms may occur before signs can be detected but in the absence of symptoms any signs are less likely to be important.

2. A careful neurological examination will usually enable the examiner to develop a sensible differential diagnosis.

3. The methodical approach that characterises the skilled neurological examination helps define the anatomical site of the abnormality.

4. Note the distribution of signs and look particularly for asymmetrical abnormalities.

5. Tendon reflexes can be absent in health but may indicate an abnormality in the sensory or motor system. An extensor plantar reflex which is reproducible is never normal (except in infants).

CHAPTER 6

The eyes and ears

Out vile jelly! Where is thy lustre now?

WILLIAM SHAKESPEARE (1564–1616)

The examination of the eyes and ears is important for any medical patient because these small parts of the body may be involved in neurological or systemic disease:

 EYES

METHOD

Sit the patient at the edge of the bed facing the examiner.
Inspect while standing well back from the patient for:

— **ptosis** (drooping of one or both upper eyelids)

— **colour of the sclerae:**

  a. yellow (deposits of bilirubin in jaundice)

  b. blue (which may be due to osteogenesis imperfecta, because the thin sclerae allow the choroidal pigment to show through)

  c. red (**iritis** which causes central inflammation or **conjunctivitis** which causes more peripheral inflammation often with pus), or subconjunctival haemorrhage as a result of trauma

  d. scleral pallor, which occurs in anaemia.

Look from behind and above the patient for **exophthalmos**, which is prominence of the eyes. If there is actual protrusion of the eyes from the orbits, this is called **proptosis**. This is best detected by looking at the eyes from above the forehead; protrusion beyond the supra-orbital ridge is abnormal. If exophthalmos is present examine specifically for thyroid eye disease: lid lag (the patient follows the examiner's finger as it descends — the upper lid lags behind the pupil), chemosis (oedema of the bulbar conjunctiva), corneal ulceration and ophthalmoplegia (weakness of upward gaze; see Chapter 5).

Proceed then as for the cranial nerve examination (page 138) — that is, testing visual acuity, visual fields (Figure 5.3) and pupillary responses to light and accommodation.

Test the **eye movements** (page 139 and Figure 6.1) Look also for fatiguability of eye muscles by asking the patient to look up at the hat pin for about half a minute. In myasthenia gravis the muscles tire and the eyelids begin to droop.

Test the **corneal reflex** (page 142). Consider the possibility that the patient may have a glass eye. This should be suspected if visual acuity is zero in one eye and no pupillary reaction is apparent. Attempts to examine and interpret the fundus of a glass eye will amuse the patient but are always unsuccessful.

HORNER'S SYNDROME

Interruption of the sympathetic innervation of the eye at any point results in Horner's syndrome. This causes **partial ptosis** (as sympathetic fibres supply the smooth muscle of both eyelids) and a **constricted pupil** (because of an unbalanced parasympathetic action) which reacts normally to light. The affected eye appears less prominent than the normal one (enophthalmos) and there is reduced sweating on the forehead on the affected side (anhydrosis).

OPHTHALMOSCOPY

Begin by examining the cornea.

The examiner should use the right eye to examine the patient's right eye and vice versa. Turn the ophthalmoscope lens to +20

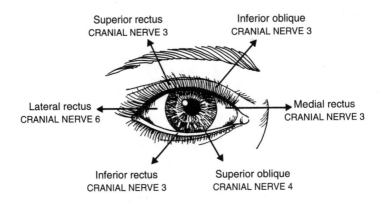

FIGURE 6.1 Eye movements, muscles and innervation.

and examine the cornea from about 20 cm away from the patient. Look particularly for corneal ulceration. Turn the lens gradually down to 0 while moving closer to the patient. Structures including the lens, humour and then the retina at increasing distance into the eye will swim into focus. A drop of sterile fluoroscein will stain corneal ulcers.

Examine the retinas. Focus on one of the retinal arteries and follow it in to the optic disc. The normal disc is round and paler than the surrounding retina. The margin of the disc is usually sharply outlined but will appear blurred if there is optic atrophy (the disc is also pale) or papilloedema (suggesting raised intracranial pressure). Look at the rest of the retinas for the retinal changes of **diabetes mellitus** or **hypertension**.

There are two main types of retinal change in **diabetes**; non-proliferative and proliferative. Non-proliferative changes include: (i) two types of haemorrhages — **dot haemorrhages** which occur in the inner retinal layers, and **blot haemorrhages** which are larger and which occur more superficially in the nerve fibre layer; (ii) **microaneurysms** which are due to vessel wall damage; and (iii) two types of exudates — **hard exudates** which have straight edges and **soft exudates** (cotton wool spots) which have a fluffy appearance. Proliferative changes include new vessel formation which can lead to retinal detachment or vitreous haemorrhage.

Hypertensive changes can be classified from grades 1 to 4:

- Grade 1 — 'silver wiring' of the arteries only (sclerosis of the vessel wall reduces its transparency so that the central light streak becomes broader and shinier).

- Grade 2 — silver wiring of arteries plus arteriovenous nipping or nicking (indentation or deflection of the veins where they are crossed by the arteries).

- Grade 3 — grade 2 plus haemorrhages (flame shaped) and exudates (soft — cotton wool spots due to ischaemia, or hard — lipid residues from leaking vessels).

- Grade 4 — grade 3 changes plus papilloedema (page 169). It is important to describe the changes present rather than just give a grade.

Inspect carefully for **central retinal artery occlusion** where the whole fundus appears milky-white because of retinal oedema, and the arteries become greatly reduced in diameter.

Central retinal vein thrombosis causes tortuous retinal veins, and haemorrhages scattered over the whole retina, particularly occurring alongside the veins.

Retinitis pigmentosa causes a scattering of black pigment in a criss-cross pattern. This will be missed if the periphery of the retina is not examined.

THE EARS

Inspect the **outer ear** for signs of inflammation or skin disease. There may be gouty tophi, seen as nodular firm pale and non-tender chalky deposits of urate in the cartilage of the ear. If there is a history of deafness or of a painful ear, examination of the external auditory meatus and tympanic membranes with an **auroscope** (Figure 6.2) is indicated. This must also be performed if there is a discharge from the ear or if there has been a head injury.

Using the largest ear-piece that will fit comfortably in the canal, inspect both ear canals and the tympanic membranes. In young

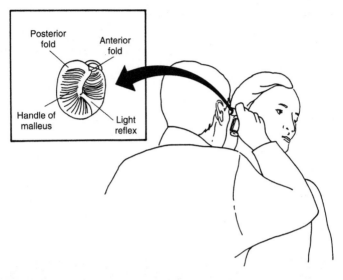

FIGURE 6.2 Use of the auroscope.

children, pulling back the pinna allows better visualisation of the tympanic membrane but in adults and older children pulling it up and back is a more effective way of straightening the canal and giving better vision. The examiner should use the right hand to pull back the patient's left pinna and vice versa. The speculum should not be forced too deeply into the ear. There is not usually tenderness present unless the meatus is inflamed. **Wax** is white or yellowish, translucent and shiny. It may obscure the view of the tympanic membrane. The normal **ear drum** is greyish and reflects light from its centre at approximately 5 or 7 o'clock (depending on the side). The drum may become pink if the middle-ear is infected, in for example, otitis media. Later it may bulge and even perforate. Blood or cerebrospinal fluid (watery clear fluid) may be seen in the meatus after a fracture of the base of the skull. If herpes zoster affects the facial nerve, there may be vesicles (fluid-filled blisters) especially on the posterior wall around the external auditory meatus.

TEST HEARING

Whisper numbers softly 60 cm away from each one of the patient's ears while the other is distracted by movement of the examiner's finger in the auditory canal. With practice the normal range of hearing is appreciated. Then perform **Rinné's** and **Weber's** tests.

1. Rinné's test: A vibrating 256 Hz tuning fork is placed on the mastoid process. When the sound is no longer heard it is moved close to the auditory meatus where, if air conduction is, as is normal, better than bone conduction, it will again be audible.

2. Weber's test: The 256 Hz fork is placed, vibrating, at the centre of the forehead. Nerve deafness causes the sound to be heard better in the normal ear but with conduction deafness the opposite occurs.

THE EYES AND EARS — HINTS

1. Important local and systemic disease will be missed unless the eyes and ears are examined as part of a general medical examination.

2. Accurate fundoscopy with the ophthalmoscope requires practice. Dilating the patient's pupils may be necessary to obtain an adequate view.

3. Subtle eye signs such as a mild Horner's syndrome will be missed unless time is taken to stand back and compare the two sides.

CHAPTER 7

The thyroid

The word 'Thyroid' comes from the Greek meaning a shield. It sits like a shield in the front of the neck.

The thyroid is a small gland which is usually unobtrusive but which exerts a powerful influence on all parts of the body. Under- or over-activity produces characteristic symptoms and signs.

 ## PRESENTING SYMPTOMS

THYROTOXICOSIS (EXCESS THYROID HORMONE PRODUCTION)

This can cause a preference for cooler weather, weight loss, increased appetite (polyphagia), palpitations (sinus tachycardia or atrial fibrillation), increased sweating, nervousness, irritability, diarrhoea, amenorrhoea, muscle weakness and exertional dyspnoea.

HYPOTHYROIDISM (MYXOEDEMA — DECREASED THYROID HORMONE PRODUCTION)

This can result in a preference for warmer weather, weight gain, lethargy, swelling of eyelids (oedema), hoarse voice, constipation and coarse dry skin.

 ## PAST HISTORY

Find out about previous surgery (e.g., thyroidectomy), and about other treatments for thyroid disease such as radio-Iodine, anti-thyroid drugs or thyroid replacement treatment.

SOCIAL HISTORY

Many of these conditions are chronic and their effect on a patient's ability to work and look after him or herself, must be assessed.

FAMILY HISTORY

There may be a history in the family of thyroid conditions. Find out where the patient grew up (there are areas of endemic goitre caused by Iodine deficiency).

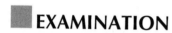 EXAMINATION

INSPECTION

Sometimes the isthmus of the normal thyroid is visible as a diffuse central swelling in the neck. Enlargement of the gland, called a goitre (Latin *guttur*, throat), should be apparent on inspection. Look at the front and sides of the neck while the patient swallows sips of water and decide if there is localised or general swelling of the gland.

Ask the patient to swallow a sip of water while you watch the swelling. Only a goitre or a thyroglossal cyst, because of their attachment to the larynx, will rise during swallowing.

Inspect the skin of the neck for scars and look for prominent veins (suggesting thoracic inlet obstruction caused by a retrosternal thyroid mass).

PALPATION

Feel systematically both lobes of the gland and its isthmus from behind the patient. Use the tips of the fingers (Figure 7.1). Note the size, shape, consistency, symmetry, tenderness, mobility and the presence of a thrill. Decide if the lower limit of the gland is palpable. Ask the patient to swallow and feel for the swelling to rise. Feel next for the cervical lymph nodes (page 120).

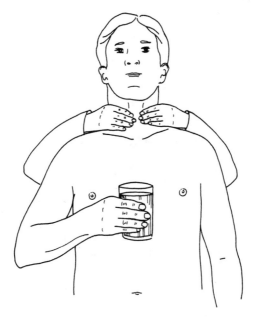

FIGURE 7.1   Palpating the thyroid.

Listen over the gland for a bruit. Listen to the patient's breathing for stridor (harsh inspiration caused by a partly occluded upper airway). If there is a goitre, apply mild compression to the lateral lobes and listen again for stridor. Percuss over the sternum. Dullness may indicate a retrosternal goitre. Ask the patient to raise their hands over their head as high as possible — if the face becomes plethoric and cyanosed this suggests thoracic inlet obstruction due to a retrosternal goitre (Pemberton's sign).

THYROTOXICOSIS

Examine a suspected case of thyrotoxicosis as follows. Look for signs of weight loss, anxiety and the frightened facies of the thyrotoxic.

Ask the patient to put out the arms and look for a fine **tremor**.

Look at the nails for **onycholysis** (Plummer's nails — separation of the distal nail from the nail bed) and for thyroid acropachy (clubbing).

Inspect for **palmar erythema** (a red appearance of the outer parts of the palms) and feel the palms for warmth and sweatiness (from sympathetic overactivity).

Take the pulse. Note the presence of sinus tachycardia or atrial fibrillation. The pulse may also have a collapsing character due to a high cardiac output.

Test for **proximal myopathy** (weakness of the muscles at the shoulders and hips) and tap the arm reflexes for abnormal **briskness**, especially in the relaxation phase.

Examine the eyes. Look for **exophthalmos** (protrusion of the eyeball out of the orbit). Then examine for **lid retraction** which is suggested by a widened palpebral fissure. Test for **lid lag** by watching for lagging of the descent of the upper lid as the patient follows the examiner's finger as it is moved at moderate speed from the upper to the lower part of the visual field. Then stand behind the patient and look over the forehead to assess for the degree of **proptosis** which is actual protrusion of the globes from the orbits.

Next look for:

1. chemosis (oedema of the conjunctivae).

2. conjunctivitis (inflammation of the conjunctivae).

3. corneal ulceration (it may be necessary to stain the cornea with fluoroscein).

4. optic atrophy (pallor of the optic disc when examined with the ophthalmoscope and due to ischaemia of the retina).

5. ophthalmoplegia (upward gaze tends to be lost first, and later convergence is weakened).

Examine for thyroid enlargement. A thrill may be present over the gland. Listen over the gland for a bruit.

Examine the heart for systolic flow murmurs and for signs of cardiac failure (Chapter 2).

Look for **pretibial myxoedema** (bilateral firm and elevated nodules and plaques on the shins which may be pink or brown).

Test for hyper-reflexia in the legs.

HYPOTHYROIDISM

Examine the patient with suspected hypothyroidism as follows. A variable number of the following signs may be present:

Look for signs of obvious mental and physical sluggishness. Note peripheral cyanosis, a cool and dry skin and the yellow skin discolouration of hypercarotenaemia (a result of reduced metabolism of carotene).

Take the pulse, which may be of small volume and slow. Tap over the flexor retinaculum at the wrist for **Tinel's sign** (tingling in the distribution of the median nerve) page 156.

Look at the face. The skin, but not the sclera, may appear yellow due to hypercarotenaemia. The skin may be generally thickened, and alopecia (loss of hair) may be present, as may vitiligo (an associated autoimmune disease).

Inspect the eyes for periorbital oedema and xanthelasma and note loss or thinning of the outer third of the eyebrows.

Ask the patient to speak and listen for coarse, croaking, slow speech.

Test for a **'hung up' ankle reflex** with the patient kneeling on a chair (the foot plantar flexes briskly when the Achilles tendon is tapped but then dorsiflexes much more slowly).

THE THYROID — HINTS

1. Not all patients with thyroid disease will have a goitre. Careful examination of the neck for the presence of a goitre is part of the routine physical examination.

2. Thyroid disease causes systemic symptoms and signs which are often of an insidious onset and may not be noticed by the patient or the relatives.

CHAPTER 8

The breasts

Breast examination should be a routine part of the general physical examination.

HISTORY

Ask if the patient has presented for a routine breast examination or whether an abnormality has been noticed. Many women examine their own breasts regularly for lumps. Other reasons for presenting include a bloody discharge from a nipple, breast pain and request for assessment because of a family history of carcinoma of the breast in first or second degree relatives.

If the patient has noticed a lump ask if it is painful (rarely the case if the lump is malignant, but consider inflammatory carcinoma). Lumps which appear just before menstruation are likely to be hormonal and benign.

The occurrence of carcinoma in the other breast in the past is a strong risk factor. Carcinoma occurring in first degree relatives is also an important risk factor. Sometimes a relative will have been identified as having a breast cancer associated gene. It is possible to test for this and its presence indicates an 85% chance of developing breast cancer.

Find out if the patient has had a previous breast biopsy. The biopsied area may feel firm or lumpy. A previous biopsy may have shown atypical ductal hyperplasia which is considered a premalignant condition. Take a hormonal history, noting the age of menarche, age of menopause, age of first full term pregnancy and whether the children were breast fed. Also ask about exogenous hormone use including the contraceptive pill. All these may influence the risk of breast cancer.

▌EXAMINATION

INSPECTION

Ask the patient to sit up with her chest fully exposed. Look at the nipples for retraction (due to **cancer** or **fibrosis**; in some patients retraction may be normal) and **Paget's disease** of the nipple (where underlying breast cancer causes a unilateral red, scaling or bleeding area).

Inspect the rest of the skin. Look for visible veins (which if unilateral suggest a cancer), skin dimpling, and for *peau d'orange* skin (where advanced breast cancer causes oedematous skin pitted by the sweat glands).

Ask the patient to raise her arms above her head. Look for tethering of the nipples or skin, a shift in the relative position of the nipples or a fixed mass distorting the breast.

Look for axillary lumps.

Ask her to rest her hands on her hips and then press her hands against her hips (the pectoral contraction manoeuvre). This accentuates areas of dimpling or fixation.

PALPATION

Examine both the supraclavicular and axillary regions for lymphadenopathy (page 119).

Ask the patient to lie down. It can be helpful to have her place her hand behind her head.

Palpation is performed gently with the palmar surface of the middle three fingers parallel to the contour of the breast. (Figure 8.1). Feel the four quadrants of each breast systematically. Start at the areola and roll the fingers over the breast tissue pressing towards the chest wall. Feel the axillary tail of the breast between your thumb and fingers (Figure 8.2).

Next feel behind the nipple for lumps and note if any fluid can be expressed: bright blood (e.g., from a duct papilloma, or more rarely a carcinoma), yellow serous (e.g., fibroadenosis) or serous fluid (e.g., early pregnancy), milky (e.g. lactation) or green fluid (e.g., mammary duct ectasia).

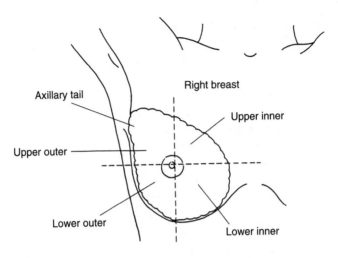

Right breast

Axillary tail

Upper inner

Upper outer

Lower outer

Lower inner

FIGURE 8.1 Examining the breast.

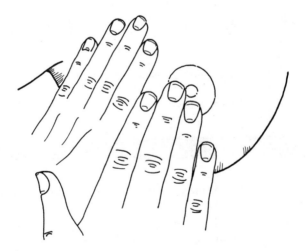

FIGURE 8.2 Feeling the axillary tail of the breast.

EVALUATION OF A BREAST LUMP

The following points need to be carefully elucidated if a lump is detected.

Position — the breast quadrant involved and proximity to the nipple.

Size, shape and consistency — a hard, irregular nodule is characteristic of carcinoma.

Tenderness — suggests an inflammatory or cystic lesion; breast cancer is usually not tender.

Fixation — mobility is determined by taking the breast between the hands and moving it over the chest wall with the arm relaxed and then with the hand pressing on the hip (to tense the pectoralis major). For lower outer quadrant lesions the arm should push against a wall in front of the patient (to tense the serratus anterior muscle). In advanced carcinoma the lump may be fixed to the chest wall.

Single or multiple lesions present — multiple nodules suggest benign cystic disease or fibroadenosis.

Lymph node enlargement — suggests metastic disease.

If carcinoma is suspected, examine for metastatic disease. Examine for a pleural effusion. Check for vertebral or other bony tenderness. Palpate for malignant hepatomegaly.

In men with true gynaecomastia a disc of breast tissue can be palpated under the areola. This is not present in men who are merely obese.

BREAST EXAMINATION — HINTS

1. **Examination of the female breasts is a routine aspect of physical examination.**

2. **The examination is not complete unless the draining lymph nodes have also been examined.**

3. **Examine for metastases if carcinoma is suspected.**

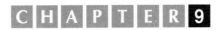

CHAPTER 9

The joints

*Rheumatism: A painful distemper supposed
to proceed from acrid humours.*

S JOHNSON, A DICTIONARY OF THE ENGLISH LANGUAGE (1775)

Joint abnormalities are commonly due to injury, inflammation or degeneration (wear and tear). Inflammatory joint conditions are often associated with abnormalities of the skin and connective tissues.

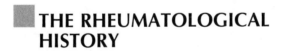

THE RHEUMATOLOGICAL HISTORY

PRESENTING SYMPTOMS (Table 9.1)

Joint Pain and Swelling

Ask the patient what joint problems have occurred. Arthralgia refers to joint pain without swelling while arthritis means both pain and swelling. Determine if one or many joints are involved, whether the symptoms are of an acute or chronic nature and whether they are getting better or worse. Patients with rheumatoid arthritis have joint symptoms which are worse after rest while those with osteo-arthritis have pain which is worse after exercise. Ask about early morning stiffness.

Ask detailed questions about the ability of the patient with arthritis to perform usual activities at home and at work (page 21).

TABLE 9.1 Rheumatological History — Major Symptoms

Joints
    Pain
    Swelling
    Morning stiffness
    Loss of function

Eyes
    Dry eyes and mouth
    Red eyes

Systemic
    Raynaud's phenomenon
    Rash, fever, fatigue, weight loss, diarrhoea, mucosal
    ulcers

Back Pain

This is a very common complaint. Musculoskeletal pain is characteristically well localised and is aggravated by movement. If there is a spinal cord lesion there may be pain that occurs in a dermatomal distribution (Chapter 5). Diseases such as osteoporosis (with crush fractures), osteomalacia or infiltration of carcinoma, leukaemia or myeloma may cause progressive and unremitting back pain. The pain may be of sudden onset if it results from the crush fracture of a vertebral body. In ankylosing spondylitis the pain is usually situated over the sacroiliac joints and lumbar spine.

Limb Pain

This can occur from disease of the musculoskeletal system (including trauma), skin, vascular system or nervous system. Pain and stiffness in the shoulders and hips in patients over the age of 50 years may be due to polymyalgia rheumatica. Bone disease such as osteomyelitis, osteomalacia, osteoporosis or tumours can cause limb pain. Inflammation of tendons (tenosynovitis) can produce local pain over the affected area.

Vascular disease may also produce pain in the limbs. Consider arterial occlusion if there has been severe pain of sudden onset. Chronic peripheral vascular disease can result in calf pain on exercise that is relieved by rest. This is called intermittent claudication. Venous thrombosis can also cause diffuse aching pain in the legs associated with swelling.

ASSOCIATED SYMPTOMS

Raynaud's Phenomenon

Raynaud's phenomenon is an abnormal vascular response of the exposed fingers (and toes) to cold; the fingers first turn white, then blue and finally become red and painful.

Dry Eyes and Mouth

Dry eyes and dry mouth are characteristic of Sjögren's syndrome which is an autoimmune disease. The dry eyes can result in conjunctivitis, keratitis and corneal ulcers.

Red Eyes

The seronegative (rheumatoid factor is not present in the blood) spondyloarthropathies and Behçet's syndrome, but not rheumatoid arthritis, may be complicated by iritis, as described on page 167.

Systemic Symptoms

Ask about fatigue, weight loss, mucosal ulcers and rashes.

PAST HISTORY

It is important to ask about any history of trauma or surgery in the past. Similarly, a history of recent infection including hepatitis, streptococcal pharyngitis, rubella, dysentery, gonorrhoea and tuberculosis may be relevant in determining the cause of arthralgia or arthritis. Inflammatory bowel disease can also result in arthritis.

SOCIAL HISTORY

Determine the patient's domestic set-up and occupation. This is particularly relevant if a chronic disabling arthritis has developed.

TREATMENT HISTORY

Document current and previous anti-arthritic medications (e.g., aspirin, other NSAIDs, gold, methotrexate, penicillamine, chloroquine, steroids). Any side effects of these drugs also need to be ascertained. Inquire about physiotherapy and joint surgery in the past.

FAMILY HISTORY

Some diseases associated with chronic arthritis run in families. For example, rheumatoid arthritis is four times as common in people who have an affected first degree relative.

THE RHEUMATOLOGICAL EXAMINATION

GENERAL INSPECTION

This gives an indication of the patient's functional disability and allows the 'spot diagnosis' of certain conditions. **Look** at the patient walking into the room and **note** apparent pain and difficulty, the posture and whether there is the need for mechanical assistance. **Observe** the pattern of joint involvement.

Position the patient for a more detailed examination, in bed undressed as far as practical. Watch for any difficulty in undressing.

THE PRINCIPLES OF JOINT EXAMINATION

Look, feel, move and measure when examining the affected joints.

1. LOOK (compare right with left), for:

- **Erythema** — redness of overlying skin which suggests active arthritis or infection of the joint.

- **Atrophy** — wasting of skin and its appendages suggests the condition is chronic.

- **Scars** — previous operations may have been performed on the joint or associated tendons (e.g., joint replacement or tendon repair).

- **Rashes** — psoriasis; this scaly silvery rash on the extensor tendons is associated with a number of types of arthritis. Vasculitis which is inflammation of small arteries causes skin (e.g., palpable purpura) and nail bed changes (e.g., linear haemorrhages) and is associated with active arthritis (e.g., rheumatoid arthritis).

- **Swelling** over the joint. This may be due to effusion (fluid accumulation within the joint space), hypertrophy or inflammation of the synovium (boggy swelling) or to bony overgrowths at the joint margins (hard swelling).

- **Deformity** — destructive arthritis causes distortion of the architecture of the area involved (e.g., the deviation of the fingers towards the ulnar side of the hand in severe rheumatoid arthritis).

- **Subluxation** — displaced parts of the joint surfaces remain partly in contact.

- **Dislocation** — loss of contact between the joint surfaces. This occurs as a result of damage to the joint surfaces and the surrounding tissues and tendons.

- **Muscle wasting** — disuse, inflammation and sometimes nerve entrapment can all be responsible for the wasting of muscles near affected joints.

2. FEEL for:

- **Warmth** — active synovitis, infection or crystal arthritis (e.g., gout) all cause increased vascularity and make the area around the affected joint warmer than normal.

- **Tenderness** — grade from I (mild discomfort) to IV (all movement of the joint causes severe pain). Joint inflammation or infection are likely causes.

- **Synovitis** — this causes a very characteristic boggy swelling which is firmer than an effusion.

- **Bony swelling** — osteophyte formation or subchondral bone thickening is very hard.

3. MOVE

- **Passive movement** — the patient is asked to relax and let the examiner move the joint in its normal anatomical directions. Note limited extension (called fixed flexion deformity) or limited flexion (fixed extension deformity).

- **Active movement** — to assess integrated joint function (e.g., hand function and gait), the patient moves the joint at the request of the examiner.

- **Stability** — the examiner attempts to move the joint gently in abnormal directions. An unstable joint can be moved in other than its usual planes of movement because of dislocation or loss of normal tendon support.

- **Joint crepitus** — a grating sensation or noise from the joint can be felt by the examiner's hand placed over the joint or tendons as the patient moves the joint; it suggests chronicity.

4. MEASURE

- **Estimate** the approximate joint angles. Movement is then recorded as the number of degrees of flexion from the anatomical position in extension (e.g., straight knee). A knee with a fixed flexion deformity may be recorded as 30° to 60°, which indicates that there is 30° of fixed flexion deformity and that flexion is limited to 60°.

- **Use a tape measure** — (i) to measure and follow serially the quadriceps muscle bulk and (ii) in examination of spinal movements (see below).

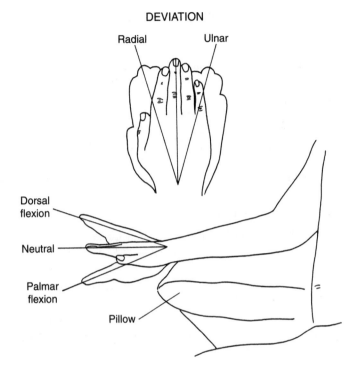

DEVIATION

Radial   Ulnar

Dorsal flexion

Neutral

Palmar flexion

Pillow

FIGURE 9.1 Movements of the hands and wrists.

EXAMINATION OF INDIVIDUAL JOINTS

The Hands and Wrists (Figure 9.1)

Sit the patient over the side of the bed and place the hands on the pillow first with the palms down.

LOOK

■ **Wrists** — Note: erythema, atrophy, scars, swelling and rashes. Also look for hollow ridges between the metacarpal bones (muscle wasting of the intrinsic muscles of the hand).

- **Metacarpophalangeal joints** — Note: skin abnormalities, swelling or deformity (ulnar deviation and volar [palmar] subluxation of the fingers).

- **Proximal interphalangeal** and **distal interphalangeal** joints — Note: skin changes and joint swelling.

- **Swan neck** deformity (flexion of proximal interphalangeal joints and hyperextension of distal interphalangeal joints) which is characteristic of rheumatoid arthritis.

- **Osteoarthritis** — here the distal interphalangeal and first carpometacarpal joints are usually swollen. **Heberden's nodes** are marginal osteophytes which lie at the base of the distal phalanx.

- **Sausage shaped fingers** (psoriatic arthropathy).

- **Nails** — **psoriatic** nail changes may be visible: pitting, onycholysis, hyperkeratosis (thickened nails), ridging and discolouration.

- **Vasculitic** changes — usually linear haemorrhages (e.g., rheumatoid arthritis).

- **Palmar surfaces** — scars (from tendon repairs or transfers), palmar erythema, and muscle wasting of the thenar or hypothenar eminences.

FEEL AND MOVE

Feel with the two thumbs at the wrists for synovitis and effusions. Note tenderness, limitation of movement or joint crepitus. Go on now to the metacarpophalangeal joints. Flex the metacarpophalangeal joint with the proximal phalanx held between the thumb and forefinger, then rock the joint backwards and forwards. Considerable movement may be present when ligamentous laxity or subluxation is present.

Palpate the proximal and distal interphalangeal joints for tenderness and swelling. Bony swelling is hard and due to the presence of osteophytes.

Test for **palmar tendon crepitus** and the presence of a **trigger finger**. The palmar aspects of the examiner's fingers are placed against the palm of the patient's hand while he or she flexes and extends the metacarpophalangeal joints. Tap over the flexor retinaculum (Tinel's sign) which lies at the proximal part of the palm. This may cause paraesthesiae (pins and needles) in the distribution of the median nerve, when thickening of the flexor retinaculum has entrapped the nerve in the carpal tunnel.

Feel for the **subcutaneous nodules** of rheumatoid arthritis near the elbows.

FUNCTION

- **Grip strength** is tested by getting the patient to squeeze two of the examiner's fingers.

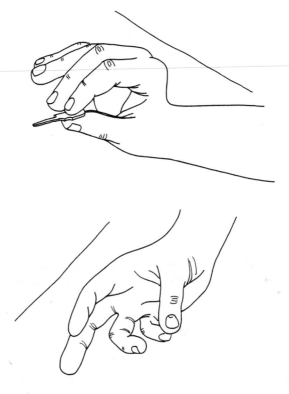

FIGURE 9.2 The key grip and testing opposition strength.

- **Key grip** (Figure 9.2) is the grip with which a key is held between the pulps of the thumb and forefinger.

- **Opposition strength** (Figure 9.2) is where the patient opposes the thumb and little finger and the difficulty with which these can be forced apart is assessed.

- **A practical test**, such as asking the patient to undo a button or write with a pen, should be performed.

The Elbows (Figure 9.3)

- **Look** for a joint effusion (a swelling on either side of the olecranon). Discrete swellings over the olecranon may be due to rheumatoid nodules (firm swellings that may be tender and are attached to deeper structures), gouty tophi or an enlarged olecranon bursa.

- **Feel** for tenderness, particularly over the epicondyles. Rheumatoid nodules are quite hard, may be tender and are attached to underlying structures, while gouty tophi have a firm feeling and often appear yellow-coloured under the skin.

- **Move** the elbow joints. The elbow is a hinge joint movement 0° — extension, to 150° — flexion.

The Shoulders (Figure 9.3)

- **Look** at the joint. Only large effusions can be detected.

- **Feel** for tenderness and swelling.

- **Move** the joint. Test **abduction** (90°), **elevation** (180°), **adduction** (50°), **external rotation** (60°), **internal rotation** (90°), **flexion** (180°) and **extension** (65°).

The Temporomandibular Joints

- **Look** in front of the ear for swelling.

- **Feel** by placing a finger just in front of the ear while the patient opens and shuts the mouth for grating and tenderness.

SHOULDER

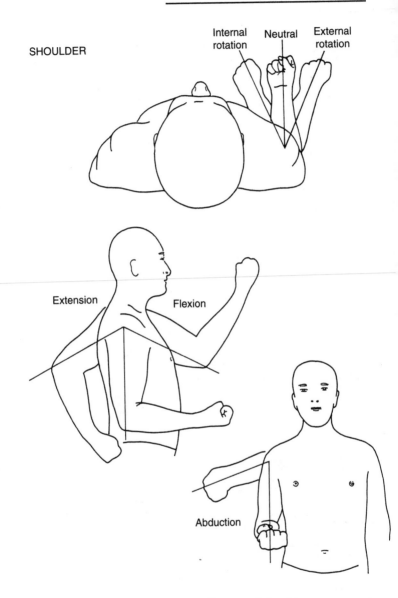

Internal rotation · Neutral · External rotation

Extension

Flexion

Abduction

FIGURE 9.3 Movements of the elbows and shoulders.

SHOULDER

In abduction:

External rotation

Internal rotation

Elevation

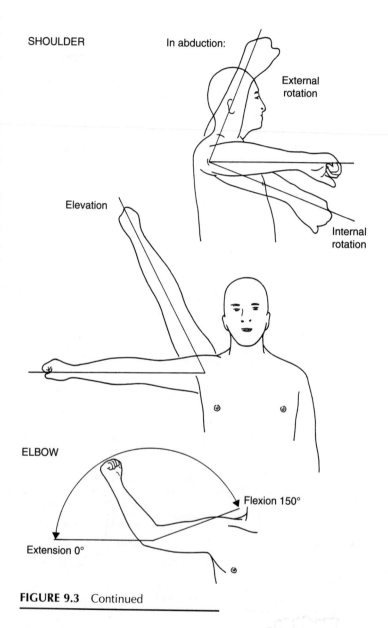

ELBOW

Flexion 150°

Extension 0°

FIGURE 9.3 Continued

NECK

Rotation

Anteroposterior

Lateral

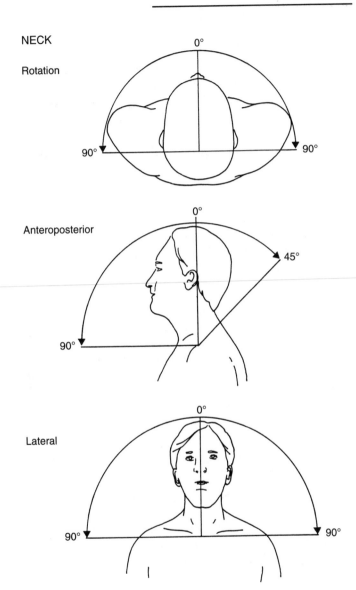

FIGURE 9.4   Movements of the neck and back.

The Neck (Figure 9.4)

- **Look** at the cervical spine while the patient is sitting up and note particularly his or her posture.
- **Movement**; test; **flexion** (45°), **extension**, (45°) **lateral bending**, (45°) and **rotation** (70°).

The Thoracolumbar Spine and Sacroiliac Joints (Figure 9.5)

To start the examination have the patient standing and clothed only in underwear.

- **Look** for deformity; loss of the normal thoracic kyphosis and lumbar lordosis (e.g., due to ankylosing spondylitis) or scoliosis, a lateral curvature.
- **Feel** each vertebral body for tenderness and palpate for muscle spasm.

Movement

Test: **flexion**, **extension**, **lateral bending** and **rotation**.
Assess **straight leg raising**, with the patient lying down, by lifting the straightened leg. This will be limited by pain in lumbar disc prolapse (page 165).

The Hips (Figure 9.6)

- **Feel** just distal to the midpoint of the inguinal ligament for joint tenderness.
- **Move** the hip joint passively with the patient lying down, first on the back.
- **Test flexion**, external and internal **rotation**, **abduction** (50°) and **adduction** (45°). Ask the patient to roll over onto the stomach and test **extension**.

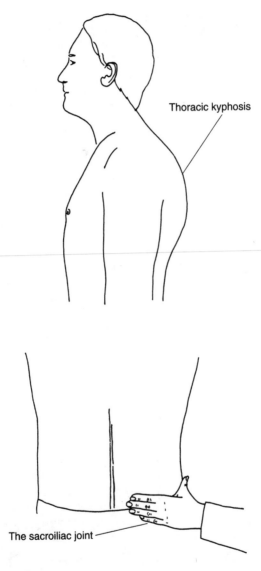

Thoracic kyphosis

The sacroiliac joint

FIGURE 9.5 The thoracolumbar spine and sacroiliac joint.

■ Ask the patient to stand now and perform the
Trendelenburg test. The patient stands first on one leg and
then on the other. Normally the non-weight-bearing hip rises,
but with proximal myopathy or hip joint disease the non-
weight-bearing side sags.

HIP

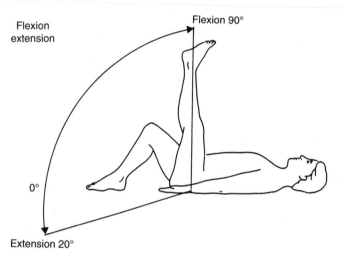

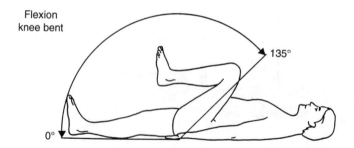

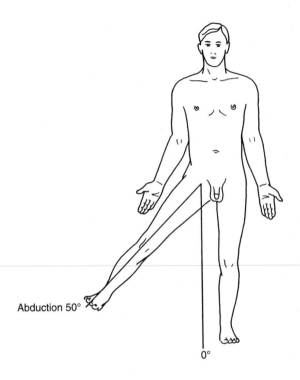

Abduction 50°

0°

Rotation

0°

45° 45°

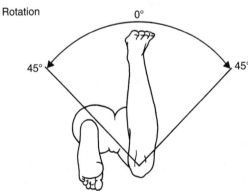

FIGURE 9.6 Movements of the hip.

The Knees (Figure 9.7)

- **Look** for quadriceps wasting and over the knees themselves for skin changes, swelling and deformity. A space will be visible under the knee if there is a permanent flexion deformity.

- **Feel** the quadriceps for wasting. Palpate over the knees for warmth and synovial swelling.

- The **patellar tap** is used to confirm the presence of large effusions. The examiner compresses the lower end of the quadriceps muscle and pushes any fluid contained in the suprapatellar bursa down and under the patella. The examiner's other hand taps down on the patella. The presence of posterior displacement of the patella followed by a tap is a sign of a significant collection.

- **Move** the joint passively.

- Test **flexion** (135°) and **extension** (5°), note the presence of crepitus.

- Test the **collateral** and **cruciate ligaments**. The lateral and medial collateral ligaments are tested by having the patient flex the knee slightly. The examiner's arm then rests along the patient's tibia and attempts lateral and medial movemants of the leg on the knee. The thigh is steadied with the other hand. Movement of more than 10° is abnormal. The cruciate ligaments are tested by flexing the patient's knee to 90°. One hand steadies the thigh while the other, placed behind the knee, attempts to produce anterior and posterior movements of the leg on the thigh.

- Finally, **stand the patient up**. Look particularly for varus (bow-leg) and valgus (knock-knee) deformity. Look and feel in the popliteal fossa for a Baker's cyst.

The Ankles and Feet

- **Look** at the skin for swelling, deformity (hallux valgus and clawing) or muscle wasting. Sausage-like deformities of the toes occur with psoriatic arthropathy, ankylosing spondylitis and Reiter's disease. Look for the nail changes that suggest psoriasis. Inspect the transverse arch of the foot and the

Flexion to 135° ↓

Extension to 5° ↑

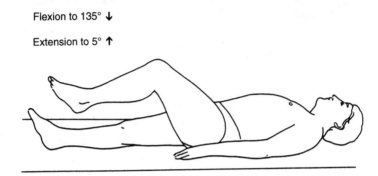

FIGURE 9.7 Movements of the knee.

longitudinal arch; these may be flattened in arthritic conditions of the foot.

- **Feel** for swelling around the lateral and medial malleoli.

- **Move** the **talar (ankle) joint**, grasping the midfoot with one hand (**dorsiflexion** and **plantar flexion**).

- With the **subtalar joint**, tenderness on movement is more important than range of movement.

- **Squeeze** the **metatarsophalangeal joints** by compressing the first and fifth metatarsals between your thumb and forefinger. Tenderness suggests inflammation.

- **Palpate** the **Achilles tendon** for rheumatoid nodules or Achilles tendonitis.

THE JOINT EXAMINATION — HINTS

1. Ask about pain and stiffness in all the joints.

2. Determine the actual joint involvement by history and confirm this on examination.

3. Always compare an affected joint with the opposite joint to ascertain the amount of abnormality.

4. Inflamed joints are characterised by redness, swelling, heat and tenderness. Impaired function is also present.

5. Functional assessment of involved joints gives important information about the clinical impact of a condition.

6. In addition to examining each joint, assess spinal movements, posture and gait.

CHAPTER 10

Examining the systems of the body

Medicine is an art, and attends to the nature and constitution of the patient, and has principles of action and reason in each case.

PLATO (427–347 BC)

Clinicians need to be thoroughly familiar with a method for examining the various systems of the body. For example, a patient who presents with symptoms of heart disease needs to be examined for the peripheral signs of heart disease as well as for abnormalities of the heart itself. A systematic approach to this is essential or signs of disease will be missed. A suggested method for the examination of the main systems is summarised in this chapter.

THE CARDIOVASCULAR SYSTEM

(Figure 10.1)

1. **Positioning the patient:** arrange for the patient to lie at 45° and make sure the chest and neck are fully exposed. Cover the breasts of a female patient with a towel or loose garment. Stand on the right side of the bed.

2. **General inspection:** stand back and look for **dyspnoea, cyanosis,** (central or peripheral blue discolouration of the skin or mucous membranes), **jaundice,** (yellow discolouration of the skin and sclerae), and **cachexia,**

(generalised muscle wasting which may be a result of cardiac failure).

3. **Hands:** pick up the patient's right hand, then left. Inspect the nails then for **clubbing**. Also look for the peripheral stigmata of infective endocarditis: **splinter haemorrhages** are common (and are also caused by trauma). Look quickly, but carefully, at each nail bed, otherwise it is easy to miss splinters. Note any **tendon xanthomata** (hyperlipidaemia). **Time** the pulse at the wrist for **rate** and **rhythm**. **Feel** for **radiofemoral** delay (which occurs in coarctation of the aorta). Pulse character is best assessed at the carotids.

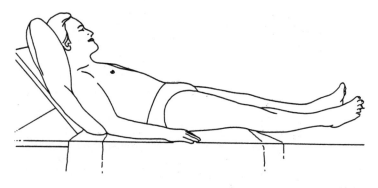

Lying at 45°

GENERAL INSPECTION

Marfan's, Turner's, Down's syndrome
Rheumatological disorders, e.g. ankylosing spondylitis (aortic regurgitation)
Acromegaly, etc.
Dyspnoea

HANDS

Radial pulses – right and left
Radiofemoral delay
Clubbing

Signs of infective endocarditis – splinter haemorrhages, Osler's nodes etc.
Peripheral cyanosis
Xanthomata

BLOOD PRESSURE

FACE

Eyes
Sclerae – pallor, jaundice
Pupils – Argyll Robertson (aortic regurgitation)
Xanthelasma

Malar flush (mitral stenosis,
pulmonary stenosis)

Mouth
Cyanosis
Palate (high arched – Marfan's)
Dentition

NECK

Jugular venous pressure
Central venous pressure height
Wave form (especially large
v waves)
Carotids – pulse character

PRAECORDIUM

Inspect
Scars – whole chest, back
Deformity
Apex beat – position,
character
Abnormal pulsations

Palpate
Apex beat – position,
character
Thrills
Abnormal impulses
NB: Beware of dextrocardia

AUSCULTATE

Heart sounds
Murmurs
Position patient
Left lateral position
Sitting forward (forced
expiratory apnoea)
NB: Palpate for thrills again after
positioning
Dynamic auscultation

Respiratory phases
Valsalva
Exercise (isometric, e.g. hand
grip)
Standing
Squatting

BACK (sitting forward)

Scars, deformity
Sacral oedema
Pleural effusion (percuss)
Left ventricular failure
(auscultate)

ABDOMEN (lying flat – 1 pillow only)

Palpate liver (pulsatile etc.)
spleen, aorta
Percuss for ascites (right heart
failure)
Femoral arteries – palpate,
auscultate

LEGS

Peripheral pulses
Cyanosis, cold limbs, trophic
changes, ulceration
(peripheral vascular disease)
Oedema
Xanthomata
Calf tenderness
Clubbing of toes

OTHER

Urine analysis (infective
endocarditis)
Fundi (endocarditis)
Temperature chart (endocarditis)

FIGURE 10.1 Cardiovascular system.

4. **The blood pressure:** measure the blood pressure with the patient lying down. An initial high reading may necessitate retaking it after the patient has spent 5 or 10 minutes calming down. If there are symptoms of postural dizziness or loss of blood is suspected, the blood pressure should also be measured while the patient stands (to assess for postural hypotension).

5. **The face:** look at the eyes again for **jaundice** (e.g., due to haemolysis caused by a prosthetic valve) or **conjunctival pallor** (anaemia) and eyelid **xanthelasma** (hyperlipidaemia). You may also notice the classical **mitral facies** (bluish-red malar discolouration of mitral stenosis). Then **inspect** the mouth, using a torch, for the state of the teeth and gums (risk of endocarditis). Look at the tongue or lips for central cyanosis.

6. **The neck:** here the **jugular venous pressure** (JVP) must be assessed for height and character and the presence of **a** and **v waves**. Use the right internal jugular vein for this evaluation. This vein runs in the line between the angle of the jaw and the suprasternal notch. Look for a paradoxical rise with inspiration (Kussmaul's sign). **Feel** each carotid pulse separately. Assess the pulse **character**.

7. **The praecordium:** (i) **Inspection**. **Look** for **scars**, **deformity**, site of the **apex beat** and visible pulsations. (ii) **Palpation**. **Feel** for the position of the **apex beat**. Count down the correct number of interspaces. The normal position is the fifth left intercostal space, 1 cm medial to the midclavicular line. The **character** of the apex beat should be noted (**pressure-loaded**, **volume-loaded**, **dyskinetic**, **tapping** or **double** or **triple** apical impulse). Feel now for an apical thrill, and if it is present, time it (systolic or diastolic or both). Then **palpate** with the heel of your hand for a left **parasternal impulse** (which indicates right ventricular enlargement or left atrial enlargement) and for thrills. Now **feel** at the base of the heart for a **palpable pulmonary component** of the second heart sound (P2) and for **aortic thrills**. Percussion is unnecessary. (iii) **Auscultation**. Begin in the mitral area with first the bell and then the diaphragm. Listen for each component of the cardiac cycle separately.

8. **Identify** the **first** and **second** heart sounds and decide if they are of normal intensity and whether the second heart sound is normally split. Now **listen** for extra heart sounds and for murmurs. More than one abnormality may be present. Repeat the approach at the left sternal edge and then the base of the heart (aortic and pulmonary areas). **Time** each part of the cycle with the carotid pulse. If a murmur is present work out its timing, loudness and the effect of dynamic manoeuvres on it.

9. **Reposition** the patient. First put him or her in the left lateral position. Again feel the apex beat for **character** (particularly tapping) and **auscultate**. **Sit** the patient up and **palpate** for **thrills** (with the patient in full expiration) at the left sternal edge and base. Then listen in those areas, particularly for **aortic regurgitation.** Dynamic auscultation should always be done if there is any doubt about the diagnosis of a systolic murmur. The **Valsalva manoeuvre** should be performed whenever there is a pure systolic murmur.

10. **The back: Percuss** the back of the chest to exclude a **pleural effusion** (e.g., due to **left ventricular failure**), and **auscultate** for inspiratory crackles (**left ventricular failure**). If there is a radiofemoral delay, also listen for a **coarctation** murmur over the back. **Feel** for sacral oedema.

11. **The abdomen:** Next **lie** the patient flat and examine the abdomen properly for **hepatomegaly** (e.g., from **right ventricular failure**) and a **pulsatile liver** (**tricuspid regurgitation**). **Feel** for **splenomegaly** (e.g., endocarditis) and an **aortic aneurysm**. **Palpate** both femoral arteries and **auscultate** here for bruits.

12. **Peripheral pulses:** Examine all the peripheral pulses (popliteal, dorsalis pedis and posterior tibial). **Look** for signs of **peripheral vascular disease**, peripheral oedema, clubbing of the toes, Achilles tendon **xanthomata** and stigmata of **infective endocarditis.**

13. **The fundi: Examine** for hypertensive changes, and **Roth's spots** (endocarditis).

14. **The urine: Examine** for haematuria (e.g., endocarditis).

15. **Take** the temperature (e.g., endocarditis or other infection).

Sitting up

GENERAL INSPECTION

Sputum mug contents (blood, pus, etc)

Type of cough

Rate and depth of respiration, and breathing pattern at rest

Accessory muscles of respiration

HANDS

Clubbing

Cyanosis (peripheral)

Nicotine staining

Wasting, weakness – finger abduction and adduction (lung cancer involving the brachial plexus)

Wrist tenderness (hypertrophic pulmonary osteoarthropathy)

Pulse (tachycardia; pulses paradoxus)

Flapping tremor (CO_2 narcosis)

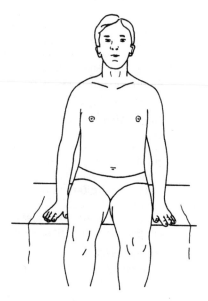

FACE

Eyes – Horner's syndrome (apical lung cancer), anaemia

Mouth – central cyanosis

Voice – hoarseness (recurrent aryngeal nerve palsy)

TRACHEA

CHEST POSTERIORLY

Inspect
    Shape of chest and spine
    Scars
    Prominent veins (determine
        direction of flow)

Palpate
    Cervical lymph nodes
    Expansion
    Vocal fremitus

Percuss
    Supraclavicular region
    Back
    Axillae
    Tidal percussion (diaphragm
        paralysis)

Auscultate

Breath sounds

Adventitious sounds

Vocal resonance

CHEST ANTERIORLY

Inspect
    Radiotherapy marks, other
        signs as noted above

Palpate
    Supraclavicular nodes
    Expansion
    Vocal fremitus
    Apex beat

Percuss

Auscultate

Pemberton's sign (superior vena
    cava obstruction)

CARDIOVASCULAR SYSTEM

(Lying at 45°)

Jugular venous pressure
    (SVC obstruction, etc.)

Cor pulmonale

FORCED EXPIRATORY TIME

OTHER

Lower limbs – oedema, cyanosis

Breasts

Temperature chart (infection)

Evidence of malignancy or
    pleural effusion: examine the
    breasts, abdomen, rectum,
    lymph nodes, etc.

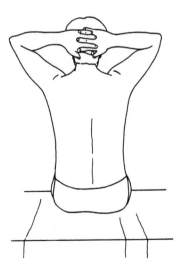

FIGURE 10.2   Respiratory system.

THE RESPIRATORY SYSTEM

(Figure 10.2)

1. **Position** the patient, undressed to the waist and sitting over the side of the bed.

2. **Inspect**, while standing back, for tachypnoea at rest and any obvious asymmetry of movement. Count the respiratory rate. Look for the use of the accessory muscles of respiration, and any intercostal indrawing of the lower rib spaces anteriorly (an important sign of emphysema). Cachexia should also be noted (e.g., malignancy). Look around the room for the all-important sputum mug and ask to see its contents.

3. **Pick up** the hands. Look for **clubbing**, peripheral **cyanosis**, **nicotine (tar) staining** and **pallor** of the palmar creases suggesting anaemia. Note any **wasting** of the small muscles of the hands (e.g., lung cancer involving the brachial plexus). Palpate the wrists for tenderness (hypertrophic pulmonary osteoarthropathy). Examine for the flapping tremor of CO_2 narcosis.

4. **Inspect** the face. Look closely at the eyes for **constriction** of the pupils and **ptosis** (Horner's syndrome from an apical lung cancer). **Inspect** the tongue for central cyanosis.

5. **Palpate** the position of the trachea. If the trachea is displaced, concentrate on the upper lobes for physical signs. Also note the presence of a tracheal tug (downward movement of the trachea with each inspiration which indicates severe airflow obstruction). Now ask the patient to speak (hoarseness which may be caused by recurrent laryngeal nerve palsy) and then cough and note whether this is a **loose cough**, a **dry cough**, or a **bovine cough**.

6. **Examine the chest**. You may wish to examine the front first, or go to the back to start. The advantage of the latter is that there are often more signs there, unless the trachea is obviously displaced. If you start at the back: **Inspect** the back. Look for kyphoscoliosis and signs of ankylosing spondylitis (that may cause decreased chest expansion and upper lobe fibrosis). Look for thoracotomy scars.

7. **Palpate** first from behind for the cervical nodes. Then examine for expansion — first **upper lobe expansion**, which is best assessed by looking over the patient's shoulders at clavicular movement during moderate respiration. The affected side will show a delay or decreased movement. Then examine **lower lobe expansion** by palpation. Note **asymmetry** and reduction of movement.

8. **Ask** the patient to bring the elbows together in the front to move the scapulae out of the way. Examine for **vocal fremitus**, then percuss the back of the chest.

9. **Auscultate the chest**. Note **breath sounds** (whether **normal** or **bronchial**) and their intensity (**normal** or **reduced**). Listen for **adventitious** sounds (**crackles** and **wheezes**). Finally examine for **vocal resonance**. If a localised abnormality is found, try to determine the abnormal lobe and segment.

10. **Return to the front** of the chest. Inspect again for chest deformity, radiotherapy changes and scars. Palpate the supraclavicular nodes carefully. Then proceed with percussion and auscultation as before. Listen high up in the axillae too. Before leaving the chest feel the **axillary nodes** and examine the **breasts** properly.

11. **Lie the patient down** at 45° and measure the **jugular venous pressure**. Then examine the **praecordium** for signs of **cor pulmonale** (a prominent parasternal impulse, a loud pulmonary component of the second heart sound and sometimes a right ventricular third or fourth heart and a murmur of tricuspid regurgitation). Finally examine the **liver** (e.g., enlarged because of ptosis or metastatic cancer, or pulsatile due to tricuspid regurgitation) and take the **temperature**.

THE GASTROINTESTINAL SYSTEM

(Figure 10.3)

1. **Position** the patient correctly with one pillow for the head and complete exposure of the abdomen.

2. **Look**, while standing back, at the general appearance and for obvious signs of chronic liver disease.

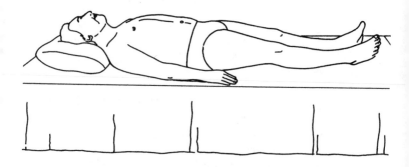

Lying flat (1 pillow)

GENERAL INSPECTION

Jaundice (liver disease)

Pigmentation
  (haemochromotosis,
  Whipple's disease)

Xanthomata (chronic
  cholestasis)

Mental state (encalopathy)

HANDS

Nails

– Clubbing

– Leuconychia

Palmar erythema

Dupuytren's contractures
  (alcohol)

Arthropathy

Hepatic flap

ARMS

Spider naevi

Bruising

Wasting

Scratch marks (chronic
  cholestasis)

FACE

Eyes – Sclera: jaundice,
        anaemia, iritis

     – Cornea: Kayser-Fleischer
        rings (Wilson's disease)

Parotids (alcohol)

Mouth – Breath: fetor hepaticus

      – Lips: stomatitis,
        leucoplakia, ulceration,
        localised pigmentation
        (Peutz-Jeghers
        syndrome),

telangiectasia (hereditary haemorrhagic telangiectasia)
- Gums: gingivitis, bleeding, hypertrophy, pigmentation, monilia
- Tongue: atrophic glossitis, leucoplakia, ulceration

CERVICAL/AXILLARY LYMPH NODES

CHEST

Gynaecomastia

Spider naevi

Body hair

ABDOMEN

Inspect

Scars

Distension

Prominent veins – determine direction of flow (caput Medusae; IVC obstruction)

Striae

Bruising

Pigmentation

Localised masses

Visible peristalsis

Papate

Superficial palpation – tenderness, rigidity, outline of any mass

Deep palpation – organomegaly (liver, spleen, kidney), abnormal masses

Roll on to right side (spleen)

Percuss

Viscera outline

Ascites – shifting dullness

Auscultate

Bowel sounds

Bruits, hums

Rubs

GROIN

Genitalia

Lymph nodes

Hernial orifices (standing up)

LEGS

Bruising

Oedema

Neurological signs (alcohol)

OTHER

Rectal examination (PR) – inspect (fistulae, tags, blood, mucus), palpate (masses)

Urine analysis (bile)

Blood pressure (renal disease)

Cardiovascular system (cardiomyopathy, cardiac failure)

Temperature chart (infection)

FIGURE 10.3 Gastrointestinal system.

3. **Pick up** the hands. Ask the patient to extend the arms and hands and look for **asterixis**. Look also at the nails for **clubbing** and for **liver (white) nails**. Note the presence of **palmar erythema** or **Dupuytren's contractures**.

4. **Look now** at the arms for bruising, scratch marks, **spider naevi** and proximal muscle wasting.

5. **Go to the face.** Note any scleral changes (e.g., **jaundice**, **anaemia**) or **iritis**. Feel for parotid enlargement, then inspect the mouth with a torch and spatula for **angular stomatitis**. Smell the breath for **fetor hepaticus**.

6. **Look now at the chest** for **spider naevi** and in men for **gynaecomastia** and loss of body hair.

7. **Inspect the abdomen** from the side, squatting to the patient's level. Large masses may be visible. Ask the patient to take slow deep breaths and look for the outlines of the liver, spleen and gall bladder. If distended, note whether central, peripheral or flank.

8. **Palpate lightly** in each region for **masses**, having asked first if any area is particularly tender. This will avoid causing pain and may provide a clue to sites of possible pathology. Next **palpate more deeply** in each region, then feel specifically for **hepatomegaly** and **splenomegaly**. If there is hepatomegaly confirm this with **percussion** and estimate the span (normal 12–15 cm). This procedure is repeated for splenomegaly. Always roll the patient onto the right side and palpate again if the spleen is not felt at first. Attempt now to **feel** the **kidneys** bimanually.

9. **Percuss for ascites**. If the abdomen is resonant right out to the flanks do not roll the patient over. Otherwise test for **shifting dullness**.

10. **By auscultation** note the presence of **bowel sounds**. Listen also for **bruits**, **hums** and **rubs**. Always auscultate over the liver, spleen or kidneys if these are enlarged or palpable, or any palpable **mass**.

11. **Examine the groins. Palpate** for **inguinal lymphadenopathy**. **Examine** for **hernias** by asking the patient to stand and then cough. The **testes** must be palpated.

12. **Now look** at the legs for **oedema** and **bruising**. Neurological examination of the legs may be indicated if there are signs of chronic liver disease (e.g., from alcohol abuse).

13. **If the liver is enlarged** or cirrhosis is suspected, the patient should be sat up to 45° and the jugular venous pressure estimated (to exclude right heart failure as a cause of liver disease).

14. While the patient is sitting up, **palpate** in the **supraclavicular fossae** for lymph nodes and feel over the lower back for **sacral oedema**. If ascites is present it is necessary to examine the chest for pleural effusions. If malignant disease is suspected, examine all the lymph node groups, the breasts and the lungs.

15. **A rectal examination** should be performed and specimens of the patient's vomitus or faeces should be inspected if available.

THE GENITOURINARY SYSTEM

(Figure 10.4)

1. **Lie** the patient flat in bed while making the usual general inspection. Note particularly the patient's mental state and whether there is a sallow complexion, the state of hydration and whether the patient is **hiccupping** or **hyperventilating** (possible signs of renal failure).

2. **Pick up** the patient's hands and look at the nails for **leuconychia**, white transverse lines that may occur in renal failure.

3. **Examine** the wrists and arms for vascular access sites. Assess the patency of an arteriovenous fistula by palpating for a thrill. Get the patient to hold out the hands and look for **asterixis**. Then inspect the arms for subcutaneous nodules (calcium phosphate deposits), bruising, pigmentation and scratch marks (chronic renal failure).

4. **Go on** now to the face and begin by examining the eyes for **anaemia**, (chronic renal failure). Examine the mouth for **dryness**, (dehydration) or **fetor** (uraemia). Note the

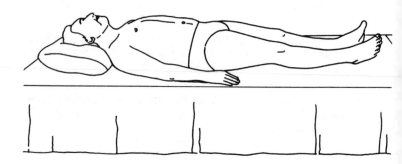

GENERAL INSPECTION

Mental state

Hyperventilation (acidosis) hiccups

Sallow complexion

Hydration

Subcutaneous nodules (calcium phosphate deposits)

HANDS

Nails – leuconychia; brown lines; distal brown arc

Vascular shunts

Asterixis

Neuropathy

ARMS

Bruising

Pigmentation

Scratch marks

Myopathy

FACE

Eyes – anaemia, jaundice, band keratopathy

Mouth – dryness, ulcers, fetor

Rash (vasculitis, etc.)

ABDOMEN

Scars – dialysis, operations

Kidneys – transplant kidney

Bladder

Liver

Lymph nodes

Ascites

Bruits

Rectal examination (prostatomegaly, bleeding)

BACK

Tenderness

Oedema

CHEST

Heart – pericarditis, failure

Lungs – infection, pulmonary oedema

LEGS

Oedema – nephrotic syndrome, cardiac failure

Bruising

Pigmentation

Scratch marks

Neuropathy

Vascular access

URINE ANALYSIS

Specific gravity, pH

Glucose – diabetes mellitus

Blood – 'nephritis', infection, stone

Protein – 'nephritis', etc.

OTHER

Blood pressure – lying not standing

Fundoscopy – hypertensive and diabetic changes, etc.

FIGURE 10.4   Genitourinary system.

presence of any vasculitic rash on the face. Note any neck scars (e.g., parathyroid surgery).

5. **Lie the patient** flat and examine the abdomen. Look for **scars** indicating peritoneal dialysis or operations including a **renal transplant**. Then examine the liver and spleen (enlargement may occur in polycystic disease). Palpate for enlarged kidneys by ballotment. **Feel** for the presence of an **abdominal aortic aneurysm. Percuss** over the bladder to detect enlargement or **ascites. Listen** for aortic and renal bruits.

6. **Sit the patient up** and palpate the back for tenderness and sacral oedema.

7. **Look at** the jugular venous pressure with the patient at 45°. Examine the heart for signs of pericarditis, pericardial effusion or cardiac failure and the lungs for pulmonary oedema.

8. **Lie** the patient down again. **Look** at the legs for oedema (due to the **nephrotic syndrome** or **cardiac failure**), bruising, pigmentation, scratch marks or the presence of gout. **Examine** for peripheral neuropathy (decreased sensation, loss of reflexes in chronic renal failure).

9. **Measure the blood pressure** with the patient lying and then standing (for **orthostatic** [postural] **hypotension**), and **perform fundoscopy** to look for hypertensive or diabetic changes.

10. **Perform** a rectal examination if indicated to feel for **prostatomegaly, frozen pelvis** or **bleeding**.

11. **Finally** urinalysis is performed testing for specific gravity, pH, glucose, blood, protein and leucocytes.

THE HAEMATOLOGICAL SYSTEM

(Figure 10.5)

1. **Position** the patient as for a gastrointestinal examination and make sure he or she is fully undressed.

2. **Look for bruising, pigmentation, cyanosis, jaundice** and **scratch marks** (suggesting pruritis due to myeloproliferative

disease or lymphoma). Look for frontal bossing and note the racial origin of the patient (e.g., for Thalassaemia).

3. **Pick up** the patient's hands. Look at the **nails** for **koilonychia** (spoon-shaped nails — iron deficiency) and the changes of **vasculitis**. Pale palmar creases may indicate **anaemia**. Evidence of **arthropathy** may be important (e.g., **rheumatoid arthritis** and **Felty's syndrome**, recurrent **haemarthroses** in bleeding disorders, secondary **gout** in myeloproliferative disorders).

4. **Examine** the **epitrochlear** nodes. Note any bruising on the arms. Remember **petechiae** are pinhead haemorrhages, while **ecchymoses** are larger bruises. Palpable purpura indicates a vasculitis.

5. **Go to** the axillae and palpate the **axillary** nodes. There are five main areas: **central**, **lateral** (above and lateral), **pectoral** (most medial), **infraclavicular** (apical) and **subscapular** (most inferior).

6. **Look** at the face. Inspecting the eyes, note jaundice, pallor or haemorrhage of the sclerae, and the injected sclerae of **polycythaemia**.

7. **Examine** the mouth. Note gum **hypertrophy** (e.g., from acute monocytic leukaemia or scurvy), ulceration, infection, haemorrhage, **atrophic glossitis** (e.g., from iron deficiency, or vitamin B_{12} or folate deficiency) and angular stomatitis. Look for tonsillar and adenoid enlargement (e.g., leukaemia).

8. **Sit** the patient up. Examine the **cervical** nodes from behind: **submental**, **submandibular**, **jugular** chain, **posterior triangle**, **postauricular**, **preauricular** and **occipital**. Then feel the **supraclavicular** area from the front. Tap the spine with your fist for **bony tenderness** (which may be caused by an enlarging marrow — e.g., in myeloma or carcinoma). Press gently on the sternum, clavicles and shoulders for bony tenderness.

9. **Lie** the patient flat again. Examine the abdomen. Don't forget to feel the testes, and to perform a rectal and pelvic examination (for tumour or bleeding). Spring the hips for pelvic tenderness.

10. **Examine** the legs. Note particularly **leg ulcers**. Examine the legs from a neurological aspect, for **peripheral neuropathy** or for evidence of vitamin B_{12} deficiency.

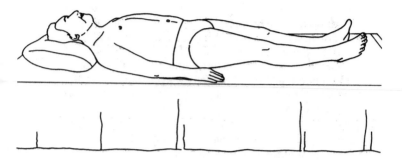

Lying flat (1 pillow)

GENERAL INSPECTION

Bruising (thrombocytopenia,
   scurvy, etc.)
   – Petechia (pinhead bleeding)
   – Ecchymoses (large bruises)
Pigmentation (lymphoma)
Rashes and infiltrative lesions
   (lymphoma)
Ulceration (neutropenia)
Cyanosis (polycythaemia)
Plethora (polycythaemia)
Jaundice (haemolysis)
Scratch marks
   (myeloproliferative diseases,
   lymphoma)
Racial origin
Pallor (anaemia)

HANDS

Nails – koilonychia, pallor
Palmar crease pallor (anaemia)
Arthropathy (haemophilia,
   secondary gout, drug
   treatment, etc.)
Pulse

EPITROCHLEAR NODES

AXILLARY NODES

FACE

Sclera – jaundice, pallor,
   conjunctival suffusion
   (polycythaemia)
Mouth – gum hyperotrophy
   (monocytic leukaemia, etc.),
   ulceration, infection,
   haemorrhage (marrow
   aplasia, etc.); atrophic
   glossitis, angular stomatitis
   (iron, vitamin deficiencies)

CERVICAL NODES (sitting up)

Palpate from behind

BONY TENDERNESS

Spine

Sternum

Clavicles

Shoulders

ABDOMEN (lying flat) and GENITALIA

Detailed examination

LEGS

Vasculitis (Henoch-Schonlein purpura – buttocks, thighs)

Bruising

Pigmentation

Ulceration (e.g. haemoglobinopathies)

Neurological signs (subacute combined degeneration, peripheral neuropathy)

OTHER

Fundi (haemorrhages, infection, etc.)

Temperature chart (infection)

Urine analysis (haematuria, bile, etc.)

Rectal and pelvic examination (blood loss)

FIGURE 10.5   Haematological system.

11. **Examine** the fundi, look at the temperature chart, and test the urine.

THE NERVOUS SYSTEM

(Figures 10.6–10.8)

1. **Handedness, orientation and speech**. Ask the patient if he or she is right or left handed. As a screening assessment, ask for the patient's name, present location and the date. Next ask the patient to name an object pointed at and have him or her point to a named object in the room (to test for dysphasia). Ask him or her to say 'British Constitution' (to test for dysarthria).

2. Neck stiffness and Kernig's Sign

3. **Cranial Nerves**. The patient should be sat over the edge of the bed. Begin by general inspection of the head and neck looking for craniotomy scars, neurofibromas, facial asymmetry, ptosis, proptosis, skew deviation of the eyes or pupil inequality.

The first nerve: examination of this is rarely required. Each nostril is tested separately using non-pungent substances in a series of sample bottles.

The second nerve: test visual acuity with the patient wearing his or her spectacles. Each eye is tested separately, while the other is covered with a small card.

Examine the visual fields by confrontation, using a hat pin. If visual acuity is very poor, the fields are mapped using the fingers. **Look** into the fundi.

The third, fourth and sixth nerves: look at the pupils, noting the shape, relative sizes and any associated **ptosis**. Use a pocket torch and shine the light from the side to gauge the reaction of the pupils to light. Assess both the **direct** and **consensual** responses. **Test accommodation** by asking the patient to look into the distance and then at the hat pin placed about 30 cm from the nose.

Assess eye movements with both eyes first, getting the patient to follow the pin in each direction. Ask about **diplopia**. Look for **failure of movement** and for **nystagmus**.

The fifth nerve: test the **corneal reflexes** gently and ask the patient if the touch of the cotton wool on the cornea can be felt.

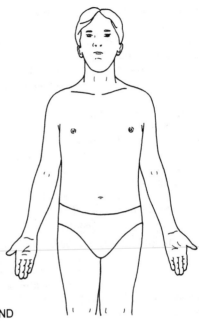

HANDEDNESS AND
CONSCIOUS LEVEL

NECK STIFFNESS AND
KERNIG'S SIGN

CRANIAL NERVES

    II Visual acuity and fields
        Fundoscopy

III IV VI Pupils and eye
        movements

    V Corneal reflexes
       Facial sensation

   VII Facial muscles

  VIII Hearing

  IX X Palate and gag
       Trapezius and
       sternomastoids
       Tongue

UPPER LIMBS

LOWER LIMBS

  Motor system
    (Tone, power, reflexes)
  Co-ordination
  Sensation

SADDLE REGION

BACK

GAIT

FIGURE 10.6 Cranial nerves.

The sensory component of this reflex is V and the motor component VII.

Test facial sensation in the three divisions: **ophthalmic, maxillary and mandibular**. **Test** pain sensation with a new pin first and map any area of sensory loss from dull to sharp. **Test** light touch as well so that **sensory dissociation** can be detected if present.

Examine the motor division of the fifth nerve by asking the patient to **clench the teeth** while you feel the masseter muscles. Then get the patient to open the mouth while you attempt to force it closed. A unilateral lesion causes the jaw to deviate towards the weak (affected) side.

Test the **jaw jerk** — with the patient's mouth open, the examiner taps with a tendon hammer one of his or her own fingers placed on the patient's chin. Brisk closure of the mouth occurs in an upper motor neurone lesion.

The seventh nerve: test the muscles of facial expression. Ask the patient to look up and wrinkle the forehead. **Look** for loss of wrinkling and feel the muscle strength by pushing down on each side. Next ask the patient to **shut the eyes** tightly and compare the two sides. Tell the patient to **grin** and compare the nasolabial grooves.

The eighth nerve: whisper softly a number 60 cm away from each ear. Perform **Rinné's** and **Weber's** tests with a 256 Hz tuning fork if there is deafness. **Examine** the external auditory canals and the eardrums if this is indicated.

The ninth and tenth nerves: look at the palate and note any uvular displacement. **Ask** the patient to say 'ah' and look for symmetrical movement of the soft palate. **Test** gently for a **gag reflex** (the ninth nerve is the sensory component and the tenth nerve the motor component). **Ask** the patient to **speak** to assess hoarseness, and to cough and swallow.

The twelfth nerve: while examining the mouth inspect the tongue for wasting and fasciculation. Next ask the patient to protrude the tongue. Unilateral paralysis results in deviation of the tongue towards the paralysed side.

The eleventh nerve: ask the patient to shrug the shoulders, and feel the **trapezius** while pushing the shoulders down. Then ask the patient to turn the head against resistance and also feel the bulk of the **sternomastoid**.

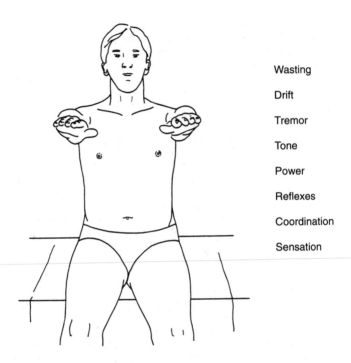

Wasting

Drift

Tremor

Tone

Power

Reflexes

Coordination

Sensation

FIGURE 10.7 Upper limbs.

Then examine the skull and auscultate for carotid bruits.

4. Upper limbs (Figure 10.7). **Ask** the patient to sit over the side of the bed facing you. Examine the **motor system** systematically every time. **Inspect** first for wasting and fasciculations.

Ask the patient to hold both hands out with the arms extended and to close the eyes. Look for **drifting** of one or both arms (caused by an upper motor neurone weakness, a cerebellar lesion or posterior column loss).

Also **note** any **tremor**, or **pseudoathetosis** due to proprioceptive loss. **Feel the muscle bulk** next and note any muscle tenderness. **Test tone** at the wrists and elbows by passively moving the joints at varying velocities. **Assess power** at the shoulders, elbows, wrists and fingers.

If indicated, test for an ulnar nerve lesion (Froment's sign) and a median nerve lesion (pen touching test).

Examine the **reflexes**: biceps (C5, C6), triceps (C7, C8) and brachioradialis (C5, C6).

Assess coordination with finger-nose testing and look for dysdiadochokinesis and rebound.

Examine the **sensory system** after motor testing, because this can be time-consuming.

First test the **spinothalamic pathway** (pain). Start proximally and test each dermatome. Use a new pin. **Next test** the **posterior column** pathway. Use a 128 Hz tuning fork to assess vibration sense. Place the vibrating fork on a distal interphalangeal joint.

Examine proprioception with the distal interphalangeal joint of the index finger.

Test light touch with cotton wool. Touch the skin lightly (do not stroke) in each dermatome.

Feel for thickened nerves — the ulnar at the elbow, the median at the wrist and the radial at the wrist — and feel the axillae if there is evidence of a proximal lesion. Note any scars, and finally examine the neck if relevant.

5. Lower limbs (Figure 10.8). **Test** the **stance** and **gait** first if possible. Ask the patient to walk normally for a few metres and then turn around quickly and walk back. Then ask the patient to walk heel-to-toe to exclude a midline cerebellar lesion. Ask the patient to then walk on the toes (an S1 lesion will make this impossible) and then on the heels (an L4 or L5 lesion causing footdrop will make this impossible). Look for shuffling (Parkinson's disease), hemiplegia (foot is swung in an arc and remains plantar flexed), or a wide based gait (cerebellar disease). Then put the patient in bed with the legs entirely exposed. Note any **tremor**. **Feel** the **muscle bulk** of the quadriceps and run your hand up each shin, feeling for wasting of the anterior tibial muscles.

Test tone at the knees and ankles. **Test clonus** at this time at the quadriceps and at the ankle.

Assess power next at the hips, knees and ankles. **Elicit** the **reflexes**: knee (L3, L4), ankle (S1, S2) and plantar response (L5, S1, S2). Test **coordination** with the heel-shin test, toe-finger test and tapping of the feet.

Examine the sensory system as for the upper limbs: pin prick,

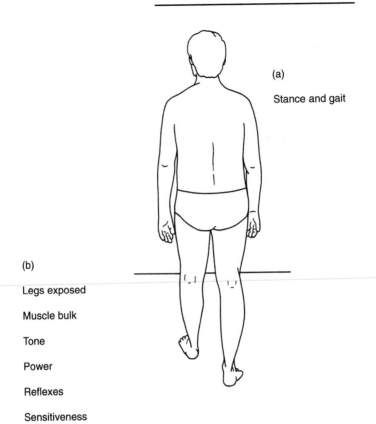

(a)

Stance and gait

(b)

Legs exposed

Muscle bulk

Tone

Power

Reflexes

Sensitiveness

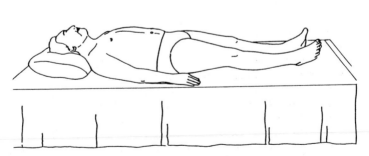

FIGURE 10.8   Lower limbs (a) walking; (b) supine.

then vibration and proprioception (beginning with the big toe) and then light touch. If there is a peripheral sensory loss, attempt to establish a sensory level on the trunk and abdomen. **Examine sensation in the saddle region** and test the anal reflex (S2, S3, S4).

Go to the back. Look for deformity, scars and neurofibromas. Palpate for tenderness over the vertebral bodies and auscultate for bruits. **Perform the straight leg raising test**.

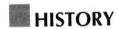

Writing and presenting the history and physical examination

Study sickness while you are well.

THOMAS FULLER (1654–1734)

It is not enough to take a history, examine a patient and make a diagnosis. The clinician must also be able to pass this information on to colleagues by means of written notes and case presentations to others involved in the patient's care.

HISTORY

PERSONAL INFORMATION

Record the name, gender and date of birth. Write down the date and time of the examination.

PRESENTING (PRINCIPAL) SYMPTOMS (PS)

A short sentence identifies the **major** symptoms and their duration; it is useful to quote the patient's own words.

HISTORY OF PRESENT ILLNESS (HPI)

Don't record every detail; rather, prepare short prose paragraphs telling the story of the illness in chronological order. Describe the characteristics of each symptom. Note why the patient presents at this time. Also, describe any past medical problems which are related to the current symptoms. Include the relevant positive and negative findings on the systems review here. If there are many seemingly unrelated problems, summarise these in an introductory paragraph and present the history of each problem in separate paragraphs. List current medications and doses and the indications for their use, if they are known, and any side effects. Finally, record your impression of the reliability of the historian and, if the patient was unable to give the history, describe who was the source.

PAST HISTORY (PH)

List in chronological order past medical problems or surgical operations, past medication use, if of relevance, and any history of allergy (particularly drug allergy). A history of blood transfusions should be noted.

SOCIAL HISTORY (SH)

Describe the patient's occupation, schooling, hobbies, marital status, family structure, personal support system, living conditions and recent travel. The number and gender of sexual partners may be relevant. Smoking, alcohol, analgesic use and other non-medical drug use should also be described.

FAMILY HISTORY (FH)

Describe causes of mortality or relevant morbidity in the first degree relatives and, if indicated, draw a family tree.

SYSTEMS REVIEW (SR)

All directly relevant information should be incorporated into the HPI or PH.

PHYSICAL EXAMINATION (PE)

Under each of the major systems, list the relevant positives and negatives using brief statements. Begin with the system involving the presenting symptoms.

PROVISIONAL DIAGNOSIS, PROBLEM LIST AND PLANS

Using a sentence or two, summarise the most important findings and then give a provisional diagnosis (PD) and list the differential diagnosis (DD).

List all the active problems that require management. Outline the diagnostic tests and therapy planned for each problem. Sign your name and then print your name and position underneath.

AN EXAMPLE OF A MEDICAL HISTORY

Personal details: Mr W Witheridge, age 72, retired botanist.

Presenting symptoms: 'I'm having more and more trouble catching my breath'. Three weeks of progressive exertional dyspnoea with 2 days of dyspnoea at rest.

History of the Presenting Illness: Mr Witheridge has had mild exertional shortness of breath for nearly 10 years but has not been physically active for several years. The current symptoms have lead to restriction of even mild exertion. He is unable to walk 50 metres on the flat. There has been no associated chest tightness or pain and no wheeze. He has spent the last 3 nights sitting up in a chair unable to breathe. He denies any ankle swelling.

There is a history of previous myocardial infarction 5 years ago but he denies any recurrence of chest pain. He has had hypertension for 30 years and control of blood pressure with drugs has been less than perfect according to him. He denies any known valvular heart disease or history of rheumatic fever. He drinks only small amounts of alcohol — 25 g a week.

He was a smoker of 25 cigarettes a day until the time of his infarct — 30 packet years. His other risk factors for ischaemic heart disease include a total cholesterol level of 6.7 mmol/L when checked at the chemist 6 months ago despite what he says is a careful diet. There is a family history of ischaemic heart disease involving his 55-year-old brother who has recently undergone coronary artery bypass grafting.

There is no history of diabetes mellitus.

There has been no previous diagnosis of asthma or of chronic airflow limitation. He has no cough.

The only other symptom has been a 10 year history of nocturia X 3. He denies other urinary tract symptoms.

His current medications are: aspirin, 100 mg daily and metoprolol (a beta-blocker), 100 mg twice a day.

Past History: Mr Witheridge's health has been good. Apart from his admission for an infarct he has only undergone an appendectomy and tonsillectomy in his youth. He was investigated for epigastric discomfort 3 years ago, was found to have an ulcer at gastroscopy and treated with a course of antibiotics, presumably for Helicobacter pylori. There has been no recurrence of these symptoms.

He has no drug allergies that he knows of and has never required a blood transfusion.

Social History: Mr Witheridge lives in retirement with his wife who is well. He has an interest in gardening and in the history of medicinal plants but no other hobbies. He has not been tempted to try medicinal plants on himself and rarely uses analgesics. He admits to a fondness for salt and drinks at least 3 L of water to help his kidneys.

He has not recently travelled overseas or been on any long car trips.

Family History: Apart from the family history of ischaemic heart disease there is no other relevant history in the family.

Physical Examination: The patient appears breathless and uncomfortable at rest.

The respiratory rate — 20/minute.

No cyanosis. No clubbing. No splinter haemorrhages. No radiofemoral delay.

Pulse rate 90/minute and regular.

Blood pressure (BP) 180/110.

Temperature 37°C.

Jugular venous pressure (JVP) not elevated.

Apex beat 2 cm displaced, dyskinetic.

Heart sounds (HS) S1 and S2 present and normal. S3 (third heart sound) present.

Pan systolic murmur grade 3/6 maximum at the apex consistent with mitral regurgitation.

Chest — Trachea in the mid line. Expansion normal right and left. Normal percussion note bilaterally. Bilateral medium basal mid inspiratory crackles and occasional expiratory rhonchi over the right and left lung fields. No areas of bronchial breathing.

Abdomen — Well healed appendix scar present. Abdomen soft, no tenderness, liver not palpable, no other masses (spleen, kidneys), no ascites. Normal bowel sounds. Rectal examination deferred (the patient was too unwell at the time of admission).

Legs — No calf tenderness. No peripheral oedema. Peripheral pulses present and equal. No visible varicose veins.

Central nervous system (CNS) — Alert and orientated. No neck stiffness.

Cranial nerves

II	Acuity and fields normal. Fundi normal.
III, IV and VI	Pupils equal, circular and concentric — react normally to light and accomodation. Eye movements normal. No nystagmus.
V	Sensation and motor function normal.
VII	Muscles of facial expression normal.
VIII	Hearing normal.
IX, X	No uvular displacement.
XI	Normal power.
XII	No fasciculation or displacement of tongue.

Upper limbs
No wasting, fasciculations, tremor.
Tone normal.

Power normal (shoulders, elbows, wrists, fingers).

Reflexes	Right	Left
Biceps	++	++
Triceps	++	++
Brachioradialis	++	++

Coordination normal.

Sensation — pain, proprioception normal.

Lower limbs

Gait normal.

No wasting.

Tone normal. No clonus.

Power normal (hips, knees, ankles).

Reflexes	Right	Left
Knee	++	++
Ankle	++	++
Plantars	↓	↓

Coordination normal.

Sensation — pain, proprioception normal.

Provisional Diagnosis: Mr Witheridge presents with the recent onset of severe dyspnoea and symptoms and signs strongly suggestive of left ventricular failure. He has no recent symptoms of angina. The aetiology of his cardiac failure is most likely, however, to be ischaemic (previous infarct) or hypertensive. He has signs of mitral regurgitation which may be secondary to cardiac failure or less likely, the cause. There is no history of chronic lung disease although he has been a smoker. The history and examination are not suggestive of pulmonary embolism.

A list of necessary investigations and, in a man as unwell as this, proposed immediate treatment, should follow.

FINAL REMARKS

He has been a doctor a year now and has had two patients, no, three, I think — yes, it was three; I attended their funerals.

MARK TWAIN (SAMUEL L CLEMENS 1835–1910)

Medical education is not completed at the Medical school; it is only begun.

WILLIAM H WELCH (1850–1934)

You should now be well on your way in your journey towards acquiring the vital clinical skills of history taking and physical examination. Despite the increasing acceleration of technological innovation in the medical field, these are the skills that you will utilise throughout your medical career. Of course, the journey will never end as learning and relearning these skills is a life-long occupation.

GOOD LUCK!

FURTHER READING

1. Talley NJ, O'Connor S. *Clinical Examination. A Systematic Guide to Physical Diagnosis.* Third edition. Sydney: MacLennan and Petty, 1996.
2. Lloyd M, Bor R. *Communication Skills for Medicine.* London: Churchill Livingstone, 1996.
3. Enelow AJ, Forde DL, Brummel-Smith K. *Interviewing and Patient Care.* Fourth edition. Melbourne: Oxford University Press, 1996.
4. Glass RD. *Diagnosis. A Brief Introduction.* Melbourne: Oxford University Press, 1996.
5. Talley NJ, O'Connor S. *Examination Medicine. A Guide to Physician Training.* Third edition. Sydney: MacLennan and Petty, 1996.
6. Munroe J, Edward C. *Macleod's Clinical Examination.* Ninth edition. Edinburgh: Churchill, 1995
7. Talley NJ, Martin CJ. (eds) *Clinical Gastroenterology: A Practical Problem-Based Approach.* Sydney: MacLennan and Petty, 1996.
8. Bickerstaff ER, Spillane JA. *Neurological Examination in Clinical Practice.* Sixth edition. Oxford: Blackwell Science, 1989.

INDEX